Before the Diagnosis:
More Stories of Life and Love Before Dementia

Compiled and Edited
by Gincy Heins

Thank you for reading these stories of life and love.

© 2022 Gincy Heins

All rights reserved. No part of this book may be reproduced or transmitted in any form or by any means, electronic or mechanical, including photocopying, recording, or by any information storage and retrieval system without permission in writing from the author or publisher.

Published by Advocacy Press, Sacramento, California

ISBN 979-8-421-03481-0

First Edition

Dedication

This book is dedicated to my loving husband, Steve, and our inspiring son, Robert. Steve is the reason I became involved in the world of Alzheimer's and Robert is my motivation to continue.

Table of Contents

Preface	v
Introduction	vi
Rich Beyond Measure, Christine Thelker	1
Alzheimer's Through the Lens of Poetry, Miriam Green	6
A Man Who Listened and Healed, Adam S Doyle	10
The Girl from Kalamazoo, Steve Field	17
The First Step in which I learn to take baby steps, Annette Januzzi Wick	20
Bettie – My Quiet but Resolute Mom, Patricia Roberts	28
In the Stillness, Susan Landeis	36
My Fiercest Fan, Susanne White	42
A Simple, Complex Man, Marianne Sciucco	47
The Last Dance, Phyllis Joly Greenberg	55
Cheese Rolls and a Punnet of Plums, Deb Bunt	61
Toodie's Story, Grant Hill	69
Toodie, The Early Years, Teri Hayes McGuire	73
A Woman of Beauty, Mary Nelson	77

Ann Hill, "Tuna Princess," Donna Corn and Karla Lucas	79
Harmony, Renée Brown Harmon, MD	82
The Tie That Binds, LeAnn Morgan Miller and Jan Morgan Alexander	89
Mother, Sister, the Best Pieces of Me, Melissa Klaeb	92
The Eighth Street Dairy, Karen Malena	96
Two Wheels and a Chocolate Bar, Elissa Boreham	103
The Traveller Extraordinaire, Elissa Boreham	107
Marathon Woman, Tony Copeland-Parker	111
The Good Soldier, Miriam Galindo	119
A Creative Helper, Jennifer Fink	129
Give Good Gifts: Lessons I Learned from My Uncle Brian, Paulette Sharkey	134
Cooking by Kindle Light, Sarah Veness	140
Index of Authors	147

Preface

It takes more than a village to create an anthology. In this case, it takes a person with an idea and a lot of people who are willing to bare their hearts and souls to share a story about a loved one. Sharing the story is the hard part. It is a leap of faith to trust that I, a stranger to most of the contributors, will edit each story carefully while keeping the story theirs. Thank you to each one of the contributors for their trust. You have done a beautiful job and I hope you are proud of your contribution to this book. Each of you has honored your loved one.

Thank you to Trish Hughes Kreis who donated her time to help me with the publishing side of the book. She was beyond understanding and encouraging as I worked to do justice to the stories.

Adam S Doyle has contributed not only an essay about his father but has donated the beautiful cover art for this book. The portrait of his father captures the essence of these stories. Thank you, Adam, for your generous gift. It sets the tone for the book and I am honored to use the painting of your father as the cover.

Introduction

When *Before the Diagnosis: Stories of Life and Love Before Dementia* was published in 2018, I thought it was a "one and done" situation. However, with over 55 million people worldwide with any type of dementia, there are a lot of stories to be shared. This book gives more people the opportunity to share their loved one's story.

The goal of this book is to remind you that people with Alzheimer's or another type of dementia are just that: people. They are so much more than the person you see in front of you. Take the time to find out more about them and appreciate them for their rich history. If you can, share some of their history with them and remind them of who they are.

It is important for all of us to remember that everyone is more than their diagnosis, whatever their diagnosis. I would love to see this book used and read by neurologists so they understand there is so much more to a patient than their diagnosis.

Thank you for reading this book. Know that your purchase of this book supports the work of Alzheimer's Orange County since 100% of the sales of the book are donated to them.

I hope this book serves as a reminder to all of us that it is important to learn our loved one's stories and share our own before it is too late.

Rich Beyond Measure
Christine Thelker

Christine Thelker is 62-years-old. She was diagnosed at 56 with early-onset vascular dementia. Christine currently lives in Vernon BC, Canada on her own with her small dog Pheobe.

Last night and for most of the morning, I have been lost in thought about how very rich I am. Those riches may not come in the ways most people measure wealth like financial status or belongings. Nonetheless, my life is rich beyond what I would have ever imagined. Yes, even living with dementia my life is rich. Oh, it's not that I have not had my share of trauma and tragedy, goodness knows I have. But had it not been for all those things I may not be in this place where I can look at and recognize how rich my life is in so many ways. I have taken adventures in Europe, many areas of the US, Mexico, Alaska, and across most of Canada, and I say most because there are still many highways and byways that I want to travel and explore. I don't want to be done yet, and most of my excursions have seen me explore areas that are off the beaten track, where I could mingle with the locals, explore their neighbourhoods, and eat in the places they eat, instead of following the tourist trail. It has created in me a richness: for people, for culture, for the natural beauty to be found in each of those places, each different, each unique, all very special.

Many of those trips were further enriched by the person or people who traveled with me. They helped create memories that will stay with me throughout my life, despite my dementia. I will look at photos and it will take me back to how I felt at that place with that person, in that moment. Those feelings can never be erased. They all bring a richness to my life that I will always be grateful for and reach from the tops of mountains to the ocean shores, the rain forests, the deserts, and grasslands.

I was fortunate enough to have my beautiful little car, which I sold when I was not allowed to drive as I could not bear to look at it sitting idle. I moved to being grateful when I was again allowed to drive and learning to love the little car I now drive, my little Mazda 3. My Mini Cooper was a special edition, iced chocolate with teal flecks in the paint. It was a lot of fun and I had a lot of great adventures with it. Richness, because I had it, richness because again I can drive and have a little car in which to do it.

My dementia has also brought many riches from the people my experiences have brought to my life, people who I would not have been likely to meet, to form friendships with, to share parts of each other's journey otherwise. Those are gifts that provide a richness that money can't buy. So although dementia takes much, it provides gifts that enrich our lives in ways we never could have expected. Beyond the devastation and gloom of being diagnosed, life becomes good, in some ways better. Maybe I had my career taken away. Maybe I have had to endure many losses and changes and challenges. But it has also brought a new perspective on life and living, on being grateful.

It brought wealth beyond what I could have imagined. Wealth in experiences like speaking at the United Nations in New York and at the Alzheimer's Disease International

Conference in Chicago, to finding the courage to write my blogs, and to write a book, with a second on the way.

My life is lived in large part in isolation, partly because of the changes since my dementia diagnosis, some by the nature of life. But in that isolation, there is also richness and things to be grateful for. Within the isolation I have learned more about myself, because without the business of life, the noise of life, I have learned to listen to my thoughts, to be in touch with my emotions and my feelings. I have learned to like, wait, no, love who I am today.

I like that I have room in my life to try to help others, to be kind and compassionate, to try to make a lasting impact on things that matter, or at least matter to me. I no longer feel less than anyone else. I have learned we are all traveling through this life and some of us are forced off of the hamster wheel. I am grateful I was one of them.

Life is lived more in the moment, with more presence, with a greater sense of feeling and gratitude. I am not saying that others don't experience that, I am just saying that for me it comes from a deeper place within. I stutter, I stumble, I make mistakes. I don't try to be perfect or do perfect. I am the most real I have ever been. That came from having my life stripped away without any say from me, forever altered. Maybe I won't like and don't want the end stage of my illness, but living with it, letting it be part and parcel of me, it doesn't control me, I don't control it, we just walk together, forever one, but we have formed a sort of friendship and respect for each other. It kicks my butt, I kick back, then we both settle into whatever is necessary for now. Right now it's kicking my butt, but in all fairness, much is triggered by the smoke and heat from all the fires occurring in 2021. It's creating a lot of inflammation and inflammation is the bad monster in my dementia world.

2021 has challenged me in ways that have been much harder than the prior year even though 2020 was a year full of changes and adjustments because of COVID-19. With COVID-19 still running rampant, with fires, heat domes, and smoke, the effects are staggering, but again I know that this too will end and I can change my focus at the other end of it all. The heat will end, the fires will end, the smoke will disappear, and COVID-19 will eventually settle into a part of our lives that is not quite so disruptive. I cannot control any of that, I can only try to manage the ways in which they impact me and do my part to ensure what I do does not negatively impact others.

I may not know the full richness this year has bestowed on me until it is long past, but I do know the richness I have already felt from it. From those near and far doing what they can to be supportive, to check, to share laughter and tears, to all of those people: they make me rich, rich in the friendships, rich in the kindness shown. I am deeply grateful to them all for being part of my life.

Right now I can honestly say I am in survival mode, trying to get through the smoke and heat and fires with as little damage as possible, although the impact on me and my dementia is increasing daily. I am feeling another level of richness which comes from the team of doctors who keep a close eye on me, who know the situation we all find ourselves in can quickly put me into a full crisis, so they monitor and I do what I can.

I am happy that I am able to see and recognize all the richness that embodies my life.

About the Author: Christine Thelker from Vernon, British Columbia, Canada describes herself as bright, fun, and adventurous and says her sense of humour has grown since her diagnosis.

Christine worked for Interior Health Authority for 13 years at various sites and loved working in dementia care and end-of-life care the most. It was here that she felt she did her best work. She was widowed at 47 and then diagnosed with vascular dementia and cerebrovascular disease at age 56. Her losses continued to accumulate starting with career, home, sense of self, confidence, and relationships with family and friends. She has since rebuilt her confidence through part-time work while writing blogs, now rents a condo, has regained her sense of self by advocating for change in how patients are treated, and has built new relationships all over the world with people who have dementia.

Her biggest achievement up to now has been to write a book about her experiences called *For This I am Grateful Living with Dementia* which is available at Amazon or at www.austinmacauley.com/us. You can read more by visiting Christine's blog at www.Chrissysjourney.com and you can find her on Facebook at Chrissy's Journey and on Twitter.

Alzheimer's Through the Lens of Poetry
Miriam Green

My mom, Naomi Cohen, was diagnosed with Alzheimer's in 2010 at the age of 69. That painful realization that we—as a family—were losing our wife, mom, and grandmother, threw us all into a panic. Over time, we learned to laugh and find joy in our newfound reality, but it was tough going. Mom was always high on life, a social butterfly with countless friends and acquaintances with whom she readily engaged in loving, meaningful conversations. Today, the situation is much different. Yet we still find that spark of love when we interact.

Brain Tangles

Dandelions
clump like tumors
in the riotous garden

of your mind. Empty diagnosis,
you insist. No one tells
the truth, not the doctors,

not your husband. Not God
behind His one-way mirrors. Sometimes
you admit you're confused.

The clock's hands read
like a foreign language.
House plants wither without

water. There's a book in the freezer,
coins in the sugar bowl.
You jam the wrong key

into the locked door and
rage when it won't open.
You wander rooms

you have already abandoned.
If there is a key, it is hidden
in the chaos of your drawers.

We sort through piles
of single socks and match
the pairs as if

we could patch your brain,
tangles that constrict
all knowledge

until even your name is lost.

In the Beginning

they ask when she was diagnosed
as if that was the beginning
as if one day one noticeable event one small
symptom drew our attention
and we could pinpoint the first moment
of her memory loss
beginning middle end
a logical concept—
we only know middle
time sliding through time
no evident trigger
no first domino
signs piling up
until they erupt into diagnosis
we try to create
beginning out of chaos
but chaos
already was

after Burton M. Wheeler

Reprinted with permission from *The Lost Kitchen: Reflections and Recipes of an Alzheimer's Caregiver*, Black Opal Books, 2019. © 2019 by Miriam Green.

About the Author: Miriam Green is the author of *The Lost Kitchen: Reflections and Recipes from an Alzheimer's Caregiver* (Black Opal Books, 2019). She writes a weekly blog at The Lost Kitchen, featuring anecdotes about her mother's Alzheimer's and related recipes. Her blog also appears on the Alzheimer's Association (alz.org/blog). She recently presented a TEDx Talk. Miriam's writing has been published in several journals, including *Guideposts Magazine* and *Daily Devotionals, Red Wolf Journal, Poet Lore, The Prose Poem Project, Ilanot Review, The Barefoot Review,* and *Poetica Magazine*. Her poem, "Mercy of a Full Womb," won the 2014 *Jewish Literary Journal's* 1st anniversary competition. Her poem, "Questions My Mother Asked, Answers My Father Gave Her," won the 2013 Reuben Rose Poetry prize. She holds an MA in Creative Writing from Bar Ilan University, and a BA from Oberlin College. You can find Miriam on LinkedIn. She can also be found as The Lost Kitchen on Facebook and Twitter. Miriam is a 30-year resident of Israel, and a mother of three.

A Man Who Listened and Healed
Adam S Doyle

James Doyle was born in New Jersey in 1943 and passed away in the early morning of December 1, 2020. During that time, he lived a full life raising four healthy children into adulthood, being an inseparable companion to his wife, and treating his patients with attention and kindness. He died at home in his sleep at age seventy-seven, following a challenging year claimed by dementia.

Soon after he retired, or quite possibly the reason he saw fit to close his office after forty-seven years, he noticed a faint fog rolling in. He was aware his memory wasn't as sharp. My dad, Dr. Jim Doyle, had great recall as to be expected of a doctor turned acupuncturist who had a diverse and ever-increasing body of knowledge. With more time on his hands, I encouraged him to entertain hobbies he'd put off, like birdwatching, which could also be a way to socialize. But he was becoming less sure of himself and more reclusive. He spoke with his friends, but with decreasing comprehension. A visit to the neurologist resulted in the diagnosis of Lewy body dementia. *Aricept* was prescribed and we tried lion's mane mushrooms. He did have us, his wife and four adult children, who were there for him. I biked over from my apartment every Saturday morning, as I'd done for years. He always had his family.

The man we loved was still accessible, but more and more locked far away inside his unresponsive body. He wandered off a few times, sneaking down the street to other parts of the neighborhood on an imagined mission. Local police brought him home. This led to social services being notified. They dropped by unannounced to assess our family home for door locks and railings we didn't have. This is the home my parents bought in 1973, where they raised four kids, which my dad maintained with his own two hands as long as he was able. We conspired to keep social services at bay for threat of taking him to their nursing home, during Covid no less. My mom and my brother Hudson took care of my dad. They did so with patience and with determination, not wanting him to be swallowed up by the system. They did an amazing, thankless job looking after him. The span of the illness lasted around a year, with the final month being the most difficult. He mercifully passed in the night while sitting on the couch. Possibly a coincidence, Hudson let us know that his phone had woken him up in the middle of the night, glowing white and burning hot to the touch. My dad's existence is now all memory, but the disease that took him was the smallest part of the life he lived.

What I can say about my dad was his genuine presence. He was present with me and my siblings when we were growing up, teaching us how to drive, each in turn on the eve of sixteen, in the family car. He was present during our calls when I was living across the country and overseas. We had good talks over the phone; he was always comforting, reassuring, and supportive. He was present every time I showed him a painting. His wide-eyed enthusiasm made me feel I'd made something special. He was generous with trusting us to do our best. He was present for my brother Nick's martial arts tests. He was there for each of his four kids, and as a family. He was a mentor in medicine to my friend Julien who became a doctor, a guide towards independent health to my friend

Laura, and a role model to my friends Nathan and Dennis on their own paths of fatherhood.

After finishing medical school he was introduced to acupuncture through Pamela during her early effort to cure her hearing loss. She said, "I was living in Washington, D.C., expecting to meet my roommate's brother, but I had no idea that I would fall in love with him. He walked into our apartment and the moment our eyes met we both saw an 'electric arc' connect between us. That was a magical moment for me, and I knew right then that we were meant to marry." They were inseparable for the next forty-seven years.

Dr. Doyle studied acupuncture in China and opened one of the first offices in New England in the 1970s. For a short time he was also president of the fledgling New England School of Acupuncture. As an early practitioner, he gave weekly lectures to educate the public on how acupuncture works. People came to him with all kinds of ailments, addiction, and health issues. His success at helping them was due to his balanced understanding of Western and Eastern medicine, as well as his inclination to ask relevant questions. He asked his patients about their diet, their habits, and if they got enough sleep. He listened to them. He would place his fingers on their wrist to feel their pulse and read the strength of their body. He deftly lifted spirits with understanding and with gentle wit. Pam managed the office and in adulthood, my brother Hudson took to the practice as well. Dr. Doyle saw thousands of patients, giving each his full attention. He listened to those under his care. He listened to passersby while on vacation. He listened to his friends and his kids whenever they needed him. If I was unwell I'd immediately be tended to, at his office or on the couch. Even from afar, he'd do what he could to make sure we would all be well soon. He was more than a doctor; he was a healer.

Caitlin, the daughter of a patient mentioned:
I remember about 20 or 25 years ago driving with my dad, a committed scientist and pro-western medicine person describing how miraculously your dad had healed him, after only a visit, and what an amazing man he thought he was. He held him in such esteem. He continued to be a hero in our family, and my mom saw him as well before he retired.

My sister Vanessa writes:
Dad was an incredibly sweet and caring man. He wanted to care for those around him whether he knew them or not. If we ever went to a party he would end up talking to a person and pulling out his needles to give them a treatment. He was such an amazing listener people just felt so comfortable talking to him. He could deeply empathize with everyone he met. He could somehow feel their pain and understand their perspective.

When we were kids he also rode motorcycles and drove a little red Lotus from the sixties. He eventually gave up the need for speed, but always kept biking. Jim and Pam biked to work year-round, rain or shine.

When he wasn't at his office he was repairing his home or fixing discarded bikes. He gathered curb-side bike parts and collected them in his basement which became his bike shop. One after another he rebuilt the bikes, then gave them away to anyone in need. In fact, anytime I had something that wasn't working, like an elf in the night, he'd fix it.

During the summer of 1998, while visiting his sister in upstate New York he was on a ride with our cousins on a quiet, residential road. He took his shirt off and hung it on the handlebars. The next thing he knew he was in the air and landed on the pavement. The shirt had caught in the front wheel. He was taken to the hospital for a broken neck. The next time I saw him at home he was wearing a halo; four rods screwed into his skull, stabilized to his upper torso atop a harness. A modern medical blessing to help his recovery, as well as a huge hassle of a contraption. He wore it for five months, all the while with levity. Humor was ever-present with Jim, ranging comfortably from dad-joke slapstick to acerbic wit. The cause of dementia is not known. We assumed it was genetic until research revealed that his brain's deterioration could have been caused by that fall, twenty-one years earlier.

Vanessa remembers:
Dad came to my high school Body/Mind class to talk about acupuncture. He asked if anyone had a cold or wasn't feeling good. He did hot cups on Mrs. Howell, the teacher. He explained that he was nervous to come and speak so he wore a rainbow sweater since it made him happy. Mrs. Howell kept reminding me all week that she still had the purple marks on her back from the hot cups.

As kids, we spent summers on Martha's Vineyard. When we got older we'd rent a lakeside house for a week in Maine, Vermont, or New Hampshire. My dad would always leave the place nicer than when we arrived. He couldn't abide ill-fitting doors or stairs with wobbly steps, so he'd fix them. He polished brass doorknobs and metal faucets to their original shine.

Vanessa recalls:
Dad had me work in the office from 8th grade through high school. I would come on Saturday mornings to answer the phones and take out needles. I think he really liked having his family all around. Mom worked there too so it was a family business. He did whatever he thought his kids needed. Each kid had very different needs and different personalities. He wanted to be sure we were all supported and felt loved. He would work on whatever interest we had to help us strengthen it. At night he would sit by my bed and ask me to read to him. I was not great at reading so I think he wanted to help me with that. He would always fall asleep and I would nudge him to ask if he was listening. He would wake back up and say yes, keep reading.

Dad's bliss was paddling along in a canoe with the dog, watching for turtles, and listening for loons. These calls always reminded him of time spent away from the city, in the embrace of nature. He loved the wistful sound of the mourning doves, writing riddles for Easter egg hunts, British mysteries, and his wife's soul-nourishing cooking. He managed to overcome prostate cancer and a broken neck, eventually recovering from both with a smile. He was a man who knew that the beauty of life was its impermanence. Jim Doyle was a source of wisdom, well-being, acceptance, and humor. We are grateful for having been his family.

He's still with us, in memory, in conversation, in our appreciation of the world, and in the breeze that carries the bird's song.

About the Author: Adam S Doyle is an artist who exhibits his paintings with galleries in the States and abroad. As a professional illustrator he works with companies including publishers, podcasts, and a variety of businesses. Heeding the call to explore, Adam lived for a time in Boston, Providence, Rome, Los Angeles, New York City, Auckland, and Hong Kong. These days he's back in his hometown of Boston, having grown more fond of quiet and the company of trees. You can see his artwork at adamsdoyle.com or you can find him on Facebook, Instagram, Twitter, and Patreon.

The Girl from Kalamazoo
Steve Field

Diane was diagnosed in 2016 with mild cognitive impairment which is slowly progressing and affects her short-term memory. Today she lives at home and enjoys doing word search books, computer solitaire, and watching television and movies. Diane always wants to go places and enjoys talking to people.

Diane was born and raised in Kalamazoo, Michigan which is located in the southwestern part of the state between Chicago and Detroit. Diane had a very happy childhood and adolescence while growing up there. She had lots of friends and a large family of aunts, uncles, and cousins. She has always been a very positive person and remains so today.

In 1942 the Glenn Miller Orchestra introduced the song "I've Got a Gal in Kalamazoo" in the musical *Orchestra Wives*. It was nominated for Best Original Song at the Academy Awards and was the #1 hit for over six weeks. That put the city in the headlines and the whole city basked in it.

When Diane meets someone she will say that they wrote a song about her and tells them she is the "Gal from Kalamazoo." As Diane grew up, she outgrew her shyness and blossomed into a more outgoing woman. She has a warm spot in her heart for all children as well as dogs and cats.

After high school, Diane enrolled in Western Michigan University and received her Bachelor's degree in special education and a Master's degree in counseling. She initially taught in Sturgis, Michigan, before teaching in Battle Creek, Michigan after we got married.

I worked in retail and met Diane when I was transferred to Kalamazoo to help open a new store. After a year there I was transferred to three more stores. We ended up reconnecting after a transfer moved me only 30 miles away.

We got married and stayed in the area for six years before I found another job and transferred to California where we presently live.

Upon our move to California, Diane found a job with Westview Services, a non-profit that helps adults with disabilities get jobs. She worked as a job coach, making sure the individuals followed all the rules and kept their jobs. One individual Diane worked with has been with McDonald's for over 30 years. Most of those years were with Diane as his job coach. He refers to Diane as his second mother when he sees her. Diane retired from Westview Services after 28 years.

We are very lucky to be soulmates who have been happily married for almost 40 years.

About the Author: Steve Field is thankful for the life-changing job transfer to Kalamazoo over 40 years ago. His life has never been the same since meeting "The Girl from Kalamazoo." When Steve isn't reading, working with his computer or taking emeritus college classes he enjoys movies, outdoor summer concerts, trying new restaurants, traveling, and California beaches.

The First Step
in which I learn to take baby steps
Annette Januzzi Wick

As an Italian American, my mother, Vincenzella, sought life's meaning through her dedication to cooking and food. When she no longer fed her family because dementia had set in, a part of her disappeared. Or so our family thought. For over six years, I sat at her side and used writing to unearth the essence of who she was. On paper and in person, she grew into the perfect state of being. After experiencing dementia for nearly ten years, in 2018, she slipped away from this world beneath a blazing June sun.

My aging parents stood on opposite sides of sliding glass doors that lead to an old sandstone building now used as a skilled rehab center. My eighty-two-year-old mother, Jean, short and mighty, planted her feet on the rubber mat. "I'm not going in." She demanded my father, Ette (pronounced *Eh-tee*), who stood at the same height as her, drive her home.

"Okay, Jean," my father said, running hands over his head where gray hairs hung on. He did as he was told.

After being at her side for the operation, I had already left town and was furious when I found out what he'd done.

My mother had begun to forget calendar appointments, doctors' orders, the names of her grandchildren. After she underwent surgery for her abdominal swelling and was released, recovery was not the only issue. The size and the emptiness of their home, as well as her care, were also problems. How could he take her home?

My parents lived in the same two-story colonial-style house close to their hometown of Lorain for over thirty years. Their soaring house was once festooned outside with *Peace on Earth* spelled out in Christmas lights along the back fence separating our yard from the highway. Inside, five children clamored for attention and the bathroom. But not anymore.

Given my father's willingness to cave in to *the boss*, as he called my mother, they were now without clear oversight and a clearer plan. Some of their grown children lived out of town, like me, or worked to balance families and jobs. I was four years into a new marriage after the death of my first husband and had three stepdaughters who joined my young son. I visited my parents less frequently and the number of children or grandchildren in the home shrank.

Surely, my parents had conversations about their long-term physical and mental health needs, I convinced myself. My father, a former business owner who staked every tomato plant at the same height, and my mother, who haunted every speck of dust that haunted her, dutifully completed Health Care Power of Attorney forms and Advanced Directives. I coerced them into filling out Vial of Life forms for emergency situations, and like a proud parent, hung the papers on their refrigerator door with the Tillamook Ice Cream magnet next to the cheeky smiles of toddler granddaughters who had the same bright, brown Italian eyes as their ancestors. I thought it was a good start. Now, I had documentation for which of my father's kidneys had been removed and which breast my mother lost. But we never addressed whether they had to move—and when.

I badgered my father across the miles of telephone wire spanning from Cincinnati to northern Ohio. "I can't believe you let Mom talk you into her not going to rehab and took her home instead. She can't get what she needs at home." How could I tell him, a man who had given everything to his family, that my mother's needs were now beyond what any one person could offer? My father couldn't do it alone and shouldn't want to try.

As adults, though maybe not in our parents' eyes, all of us children made phone calls and outright pleas for my father to admit he needed assistance. My youngest sister, Jeanne, lived nearby and had been dutifully on standby for years, but even she couldn't maintain that position forever. "We'll pay for it," I offered, knowing money was at the heart of some things that mattered to him. We were willing to pay for a cleaning person, someone to mow the **damn grass** (as my mother called the half-acre of green), rake the leaves that fell from the three silver maple trees. Someone, anyone. I lived four hours away by car—I couldn't offer myself.

"I don't want strangers in here," my father said gruffly into the brown desk phone, in the stubborn tradition associated with his generation and Italian background. I imagined him sitting in his den, surrounded by his former lives of shoe store proprietor and real estate agent. "We have lots of valuables. My stamp collection. Your mother's Lladro figures. Someone'll walk off with them. I don't want anyone else in my business."

For weeks, my four siblings and I lobbed comments and suggestions toward my father. For weeks, he tossed them aside. He played the role of martyr to one child—*What do you want me to do?*—and the role of strong dictator to the next—*I won't do it.* I often hung up the phone confused. Had I spoken to Jekyll or Hyde?

My father's short black locks had thinned and grayed over the years, coiling mostly around his lower head to keep his ears warm. I didn't know what raw emotion or information couldn't get through his head—or weakened heart valves. Over the phone, I couldn't see how his love for my mother and the shame of not being able to care for his wife might also cause him to fear the unknown. I did, however, possess the background of tending to my first husband, Devin, through his cancer diagnosis and death. I still regretted that in Devin's death, I gave more care than I did love, because that was what was required. *Do you understand that, Dad?* Here I was, the daughter, counseling him against making the same mistake I had made.

Perhaps my father felt it was his duty to provide care for his wife in the way of food, clothing and shelter. And this he was doing.

The night before my mother's operation, I had slept in the sunny yellow bedroom of my youth in my parents' home. In the age-old tradition of foraging through the kitchen for leftovers, I smelled something foul and found a roast of turkey turned blue, rotting in the refrigerator. Dish towels were left unwashed and stiff. Baggies from store-bought cold cuts were being reused to store wedges of Romano cheese. My parents must have thought salmonella had been eradicated.

And, as I told my father, "I think Mom is lonely and she could use a hair wash."

My mother once maintained a pristine home with carpeting fibers in every room standing at attention, and an unspoiled personal appearance where not a brown or graying hair lay out of place. Like my father, she was of her generation. She took pride in what little she could control. Before driving to the hospital for her operation, she halted progress at the hallway mirror to swipe on some muted red color of lipstick. And throughout her stay, she kept asking, "Where is my comb?" She looked for her flimsy comb in the plastic bin, the nightstand, and her sheets.

My father and I waited in the hard, vinyl chairs of the hospital, surrounded by the scents of sterility and reality, and grunted at her incessant questions. *Where am I? What is this?*

He looked at me with sunken brown eyes. "I should have taken your mother on more vacations." Adventuresome before marriage, my mother always wanted to travel. Over the years, she arranged family outings to center around warm temperatures, while my father pushed for more historical context in our trips. But in their later years, he preferred to stay at home, watching his pennies or his garden.

At first, I trembled at his admission. Then I'd wondered if my father's comment was a sign that he saw the future. He was ready to take that first step—admitting there was a problem.

But then he allowed my mother to walk out of therapy critical to her healing. Of course, she, too, was of an obstinate, Italian ancestry and plotted out her day with the same vision as she plotted tasks in the kitchen. She was hard to cross.

Now, following my mother's surgery, my father was trapped. At home, she forgot her ravaged body could not hold weight and lifted overflowing laundry baskets and grocery bags of flour and sugar. "At least she's doing the laundry," he said when I blew up at him over the phone, fast becoming a habit of mine. He balked again at additional help, giving more of his tired lines. "I don't want new people in the house. They'll scare your mother."

"But what would scare her more? A house on fire? An unrecognizable home? A move?" I hadn't meant to throw out a threat, so I softened. "These caregivers could also become friends." My mother was a friend gatherer, the first link in a phone chain, the first to drop a get-well card in the mail. She was a person who needed people. And she could use a friend to return the favor, one who might not fear her as she retreated to the corners of her mind, unlike her children who pressured her into doing what we wanted.

"Remember what you said about vacations, Dad? I doubt Mom will be going on too many more, but she can still retain some dignity." I didn't know how much he really respected my opinions, as we hadn't been close since I moved away after college. But I felt it was my duty to lobby for my mother. My past role as advocate for Devin might not have persuaded my father to act, but it had taught me to be the voice for decency. "And she could still have a clean home and good hair," I added as a joke.

My father and I made a deal. He would concede. So would I.

He yielded long enough for a woman named Tamara to visit and sit with my mother. We did not talk in detail about the situation. I didn't want to open the door for him to picket our pact.

One morning, I called home. Tamara answered and said my father had just left for a meeting. In the background, I heard my mother laughing as she came to the phone. "Hi, Mom. What are you up to?"

"Oh. Hi, 'Net."

For years, my mother had called me 'Net and, to my father, I was 'Net Marie. According to her, she gave her children names that could not be shortened. But Annette did lend itself to nicknames. And for years, I'd endured monikers and mispronunciations such as Nettie, Netti Spaghetti, Annie, Anita, or Janette, until one day I discovered my great-grandmother had been named *Annatonia*. I longed to be that woman instead, one with an Italian name, though *Annatonia* and *Annette* were rather close in sound.

My knees weakened at the sound of my nickname. It had taken forty years for me to find out I didn't need to be Annette or Annatonia. Suddenly, I was thrilled to be 'Net to her, to hear the lightness in her voice.

"I have a friend here," my mother continued. "And we're going to sit outside. It's so beautiful today."

"Yeah? What's it like?"

"Colors. And sun."

Living over two hundred miles away in Cincinnati, I imagined a similar fall day to the one I was experiencing while gazing out the sliding glass door of my kitchen into the stand of cottonwood trees, a crisp apple smell detected in the wash of red and orange leaves floating through the air. I puffed up my chest, hearing my mother smile in her declaration.

We didn't speak at length. I wanted her to hold fast to that sense of friendship and freedom and sunshine. I hung up and cried a little, called my youngest sister to relay the story and sobbed again.

We were all taking baby steps.

excerpted from I'll Have Some of Yours, reprinted with permission.

About the Author: Annette Januzzi Wick is a writer, speaker, and author of *I'll Have Some of Yours: What my mother taught me about dementia, cookies, music, the outside, and her life inside a care home (Three Arch Press)* and is a recipient of a 2020 National Society of Newspaper Columnists award. Visit annettejwick.com to learn more.

Bettie - My Quiet but Resolute Mom
Patricia Roberts

Bettie Pierce was officially diagnosed with Alzheimer's disease in February 2020 at the age of 80. She moved to a memory care unit in an assisted living facility in August of 2020 and was loved by all the staff. After complications from a fall in June of 2021, Bettie was lovingly cared for in hospice and passed away on July 15, 2021, at the age of 82.

My mother was late all her life, despite being one of the most responsible people I have known. My grandfather said her tardiness while she was growing up was the sole reason he would never have another two-door car. He and my grandmother grew tired of repeatedly getting out of the car and folding down the front seat so Bettie could climb in the back seat to join her younger sisters, Bonnie and Johnnie, all of them sitting in the driveway waiting for mom.

My aunt Johnnie can't remember why at that early age Bettie was always late for everything, even working in the family country store in rural Simpson County, Mississippi. The three girls would work in the store before and after school, each girl responsible for a different section. Mom from an early age handled the cash register. Johnnie said that although Mom arrived a little late she was one of the best workers you could find, always hard-working and conscientious.

Those habits stuck with Mom later in life while she was raising my brother, Charlie, and me as a single mom in Jackson, Mississippi, where I grew up. I remember the embarrassment of walking into Sunday school late every week wondering why my mom could not get us there on time like everyone else. It is only later in life that I have come to realize that Mom was late, not because of idleness, laziness, or lack of consideration for anyone else, but because she always wanted to do "one more thing" before we left. There was always something else to tend to, either in the small ranch house she purchased on a legal secretary's salary or in the vegetable garden behind the house.

My mother was smart and liked to figure things out. It really was a shame Mom never attended college. She would have had a bright future in whatever career she pursued. Unfortunately, my mom's college attendance was a casualty of my parent's failed marriage. Even though she worked so my dad could get his degree, her opportunity for higher education never came. She and my dad divorced when my brother was a year old and I was five, leaving Mom with two small children to raise alone.

During the forty years Mom worked as a legal secretary, typewriters became word processors and then evolved into computers. When all the other secretaries left for a day of training on these new gadgets, Mom stayed behind to keep the office going. Later she would study the manual and learn on her own how to operate the new equipment. At home or work, Mom always exhibited confidence that she could resolve any problem.

She operated that way in all areas of her life. She had a saying "you need to know what is wrong with you before you go to the doctor." She liked the efficiency of saving the doctor's time and her money, plus she felt like it was only common sense that you would be aware of what was happening in your own body. She would keep track of her symptoms, research all the possibilities and see if there were any practical changes she could make in her life to cure what was ailing her. If that didn't work, she would go to the doctor, having already eliminated the obvious.

This worked well all her life until in her late seventies she started having trouble putting all the pieces together. Bettie's memory started to fail her, and confusion began to creep in. A part of me thinks she did not understand what was happening, yet another part of me thinks she knew something was wrong, so seriously wrong she rejected seeing a doctor and refused to discuss the possibility. For more than a year she avoided me because I voiced concerns about her memory and would bring up going to the doctor. For the first time in my life, I saw my mom change from the practical no-nonsense woman who faced problems head-on to a secretive, defensive and angry person. How scared she must have been to feel like she was losing control when she had always succeeded in taking care of herself and her two children, and then her parents when they were elderly and could not take care of themselves.

Independence and self-reliance were important to Bettie. My mom was in a serious car accident while I was growing up which affected how she raised me and my brother. When I was an adult Bettie told me that at the time she was worried that if she passed away we would not have anyone to care for us. She decided that Charlie and I needed to know the basics of running a house, from laundry and cooking to cleaning and working in the garden and putting up food in the freezer. She talked about finances with us and my brother and I both got jobs early on, instilling in us that one needed to work for what one gets. My mom could be tough when she needed to be. We were expected to behave, say "yes ma'am" and "no sir" and not get in trouble at school. We had a curfew and she made sure we honored that and any other rules she laid down.

Although we did not have a lot of money growing up, I never felt like we were poor. Maybe it was due to one of mom's sayings that "you are as good as anybody else but not any better than anybody else" or maybe it was due to mom's creative ways of making sure we had what we needed.

Even though for many years my clothes were either homemade or were bought from the racks of the "fire sale" store I never felt deprived. I still remember Saturday afternoons perched high on a stool flipping through pattern books with mom as we looked for just the right design, then surveying all the bolts of fabric, buttons, and zippers, and finally hearing scissors slicing through the material as the saleslady cut the fabric from the bolt. That was the fun part. Then Mom got to work at night and on the weekends, meticulously pinning the pattern pieces to the fabric for cutting, hunching over a sewing machine for hours, and then hemming tiny precise stitches under lamplight by hand late into the night. How tired her eyes, back, and shoulders must have been after all that typing at work, yet she never complained. I don't recall ever feeling that my clothes were not as nice as anyone else's store-bought clothes.

My mom had a unique solution for Christmas presents when my brother and I were teenagers. Bettie could not afford to buy both of us expensive gifts at Christmas, particularly the larger ticket items that our peers were beginning to receive. Mom rotated who got the "big" present each year. One year I got a stereo and the next year my brother got a ten-speed bike and so on. I don't recall either one of us complaining and I look back now on how clever mom was to think outside of the box so her kids could have something special like their friends did without breaking the bank. I don't have the stereo anymore, but I will always remember how fair my mom was about the whole thing and how we trusted her from year to year that if this wasn't your year then next year it was your turn.

Mom loved dogs but we could only afford to have one at a time, always from the local animal rescue organization. Mom would always say "I may not have a lot of dogs, but I am going to take good care of the one I have" and she always did. From Poochie and Bogey to Rosie and Bunny, mom always had a faithful dog to cherish and love and to be adored by in return. When my dog, Lady, at the age of sixteen passed away I was heartbroken and took the day off from work. My mom offered to spend the day with me and took me to lunch. I couldn't even talk about it without sobbing but my mom knew that I could not face being alone that day. One dog lover comforting another dog lover.

One Christmas I was having problems with my dad and I was not going to see him or that side of the family for Christmas. I was a teenager, and I was upset. My mom, who never went to the movies, suggested we go to the movies on Christmas day, and I will always remember watching *Nine to Five* on the big screen, laughing and forgetting my troubles for a few hours.

Those are just a few examples of how my mom shared her love. There were no grand gestures and not a lot of flowery words. She was a quiet woman determined to take care of her children and give them what she could, no matter how hard she had to work. She paid for braces for me and my brother instead of vacations or meals out for herself. Someone once told me that she was self-conscious about her teeth (which always looked fine to me) and she wanted her kids to have beautiful smiles.

After I left for college, my mom remarried, and a new era of her life began. For so long she had devoted herself to raising Charlie and me. She never dated because she didn't have time for a social life. Bettie and her husband, Jan, enjoyed exploring with their dog in their RV, cooking, gardening, and home improvement projects. As they traveled they enjoyed the challenge of seeing if they could recreate dishes they were served at restaurants they visited. If bread pudding was a menu item my mom had to try it out. She loved experiencing all the variations that chefs came up with. Bettie and Jan dreamed one day of building a log cabin on a lot they bought on a mountaintop in North Carolina. Life got in the way and despite all the log cabin plans they pored over and all the research they did, sadly, they never got around to building their dream home.

My stepdad passed away last year after he and mom both moved to the memory-care unit at an assisted living facility. One of the few blessings of Alzheimer's is that my mom did not seem to realize Jan, her husband of thirty-nine years was gone. She seemed to think he happened to be somewhere else.

As she grew older, my mom became a frail woman, although in her eighty-two years she was always trim with a calm demeanor and a steady gaze from light blue-gray eyes. When I would tell her that her hair, which was still mostly brunette with only a smattering of gray, was cute, she would roll her eyes and say, "you've got to be kidding," deftly side-stepping an honest compliment. She was, despite Alzheimer's disease, unfailingly polite to all and would offer you the food off her plate if she was eating and you were not. Alzheimer's did not rob my mom of the manners that her parents taught her decades ago.

Without mom's example of independence, hard work, and confidence that you can figure anything out if you put your mind to it, I honestly do not believe I would have been able to handle everything that the past two years have thrown at me.

Taking care of mom, my Aunt Bonnie and for a time my stepdad, all with varying levels of dementia, has been a challenge in the pandemic while I continue to work full-time. It helps that at times I remember the gentle way she took care of her parents. I want to give the same to her, not shorting her on the level of care and dignity she deserves.

Mom worked for decades as a top-notch legal secretary every day so her children could have a better life, become independent and take advantage of opportunities that would come their way. About the time she retired from the workforce the firm moved and bought new furniture. Mom asked if I wanted the desk that she used every day for decades and of course, I said yes. I continue to use this desk as I run my own business, and in my spare time to follow my dream of writing. It is not lost on me that my mom laid the foundation for me to become who I am today by sitting at this desk and putting in long hours. As always mom figured out what had to be done, she laid her plans and worked at it every day always doing her best.

About the Author: Patricia Roberts graduated from the University of Southern Mississippi in 1985 with a degree in Paralegal Studies. She has worked in the real estate field as an abstractor (someone that examines the title to real property) and also as a title plant manager for a time in Birmingham, Alabama. She moved back to Mississippi to be with family and now runs her own abstracting business. She has always wanted to write for herself but is now focusing more on this passion and has plans for a book to help caregivers for persons with Alzheimer's navigate this stressful time. Her goal with this book is to help the people that don't know what to do to help the caregiver and make the life of the caregiver easier. You can find Patricia on Facebook or follow her on Twitter and Instagram @AisforAlz.

In the Stillness
Susan Landeis

After suffering with cognitive issues for many years, Arlene Scott was officially diagnosed with Lewy body dementia in 2010 at the age of 72. She passed away two years later from related complications, just two weeks before her 74th birthday, on Leap Day, February 29th, 2012.

In the stillness of the morning light, my mother sits in her favorite chair, gazing out the window. As she looks up at me, I see the questions in her faded blue eyes. I realize she has forgotten who I am, but I sense that her heart still remembers.

I would like to say that my mother and I had one of those close, easy relationships that some people seem to have, but it was complicated, to say the least. Perhaps, that is what makes our story so endearing.

My mother, Arlene, was a bright and beautiful, shy young woman, fresh out of beauty school when she met my father. My mother's best friend introduced her brother-in-law (my father) to my mother at a picnic, and the rest, as they say, is history!

My father worked hard to advance in his career as a civil engineer, and my mother was a dedicated wife and homemaker. They settled into married life, had three children, bought their first home, and were living the American dream.

Everything about their life seemed idyllic, that is until my mother's dark side began to emerge. Not long after my parents married, she began suffering from bouts of depression and grief. I always believed these episodes were the result of a traumatic childhood, and later on, the loss of her child just two years before I was born.

In the 1960s and 1970s, people who suffered from mental health issues were often judged and misunderstood.

Because of a lack of support and understanding, my mother suffered in silence as her depression slowly worsened.

There were times, however, when the fog lifted, and she appeared almost normal. I would come home from school and smell a delectable aroma coming from the kitchen, and I knew she had spent the afternoon baking her famous banana bread. She would greet me with a smile and offer a warm slice of bread slathered with butter. I believe the act of baking was somehow therapeutic for my mother because it always seemed to lift her spirits. It was days like this that made me want to believe there was hope for the future.

Over the years, her behavior became more erratic, resulting in angry outbursts and unpredictable mood swings. My father helplessly stood by her, but we all suffered as a family.

Unable to cope with her growing cruelty and rejection, I left home at the age of sixteen. I married at a young age, moved away, and never looked back. Throughout the years, I had very little contact with my mother, and my relationship with my parents consisted mainly of phone calls and occasional visits.

In 2006, my mother was diagnosed with Parkinson's disease. Her behavior by that time had become increasingly more bizarre, and her doctor suggested that she may be suffering from schizophrenia. I had a hard time believing this was true, but the medication he prescribed took the edge off and seemed to calm her down. My father chose to care for her as long as he could. But the disease quickly progressed, and decisions had to be made.

By 2010, it was evident that my father could no longer care for her himself. His health was beginning to suffer, and they both needed help. Even though I had a younger brother, I was the one who became the family caregiver. It was a difficult decision, given our past, but I couldn't turn my back on them. Little did I know that it would turn out to be a blessing in disguise.

When I finally got my father's health issues under control, my mother's condition only seemed to worsen. A doctor's visit revealed that she had Parkinson's related dementia, which explained some of her new symptoms. Oddly enough, her personality began to change dramatically. My mother suddenly became softer, more approachable, and our relationship began to evolve.

Sadly, the day came when my mother required more care than my father or I could give her. We made the difficult decision to place her in a care facility in my home state of Colorado, so I could continue to care for both of my parents.

At first, it felt strange having my parents living nearby, but as time went on, my mother and I developed a close bond. As old wounds began to heal, we eventually found peace, understanding, and forgiveness. I was starting to believe that I would finally have the mother I always longed to have.

Not long after her admission to the care facility, the doctor suggested further cognitive testing. It came as a surprise when the doctor told me that she believed my mother had Lewy body dementia. It was something I had never even heard of before!

I researched the disease and was astonished at the information I found. According to the National Institute on Aging, over 1 million people in the United States have been affected by Lewy body dementia. It is also the second most common type of dementia after Alzheimer's disease.

This type of dementia is typically more aggressive and mainly affects motor control, thinking, and reasoning capabilities. Some of the early symptoms include depression, distortion of reality, hallucinations, psychiatric symptoms, restlessness, aggressiveness, change in personality, and sleep disorders.

After learning all that I could about LBD, it raised some interesting questions. Could this explain some of my mother's much earlier behavior? How long had she had this disease? Since there is still very little information known about Lewy body dementia, all we could do is speculate the answers.

Dementia is a cruel disease that steals away people's minds and memories, but for us, it was a bitter-sweet journey. It was, after all, what brought my mother and me together again. It enabled us to close a significant gap in our lives, as we came full circle.

In the stillness, I can recall my mother's face and sometimes feel her presence nearby. I will always remember her strength and courage, her flaws and imperfections, and the softness that came at the end of her life. She was a woman with a place in society, in our lives, and our hearts. She was my mother, Arlene.

It is my hope that with new medical advancements and continuing advocacy, there may someday be a cure!

About the Author: Susan Landeis is a writer, author, senior care advocate, and certified nutritionist. Prior to this, she spent over twenty years in Health Information Management.

She is the author of two books. *In Search of Rainbows: A Daughter's Story of Loss, Hope, and Redemption,* is a memoir of her personal life story as a family caregiver. Her first book, *Optimal Caregiving: A Guide for Managing Senior Health and Well-being,* is a supportive and practical guide that focuses on senior care, nutrition, and self-care for the caregiver.

Susan is a wife, mother, and proud grandmother of three. She lives in the beautiful state of Oklahoma and continues to care for her father. When she is not working on her latest projects, she enjoys spending time in the great outdoors with her husband and two dogs.

Most recently, Susan has become an assistant manager for the AlzAuthors non-profit organization. A website created to connect resources with caregivers, increase awareness of Alzheimer's and dementia, and reduce the stigma of a diagnosis.

Susan Landeis' books are available on Amazon, or you can visit her website www.susanlandeis.com for more information.

My Fiercest Fan
Susanne White

Mom was diagnosed with dementia and passed in the summer of 2010, seven weeks after my father's passing. I believe she died of a broken heart.

My mother and I were at odds with each other. For years we just didn't get along. Yet even as we fought and banged heads, there was no denying we loved each other deeply. I used to think we had such a hard time because we were so different. I now know it was because we were so much alike.

When my mother was diagnosed with dementia, my immediate response was to become her caregiver. I never thought twice about it, and I never looked back. I encountered many surprises along the way but never expected to be given a chance to mend our relationship. The pain of watching her slip away from me allowed me to experience empathy that tore down the walls of resentment and anger. The healing that occurred between us was miraculous and blessed. It opened my eyes and helped me remember the mother that had given me so much. It gave me back the precious memories I had lost along the way and gratitude for the woman that taught me extraordinary lessons.

My mother's first love was killed in Air Force training maneuvers during WWII. She told me the day it happened, she was walking down the stairs in her home and faced a large mirror on the wall. She said she paused to look into it and knew right then and there he was dead. I can still see the look on her face as she told me this story. She must have been so young and heartbroken. She would later give me the ring he gave her for their engagement. His name was Teddy.

She said her faith kept her strong and a few years later she cared for my father when he came home from the war, a wounded pilot and hero. She told me they found each other through grief and survival and planned a life together.

They waited five years for me after they married. She said they had tried so hard to have a child, and it was only when she tried to let go and surrender to fate, did I arrive. I still to this day make big entrances.

Of all the lasting things she taught me and all the things I learned, two things are outstanding. The way she laughed out loud and the support she always showed for my singing, writing, and creative process. I would try my entire life to get her to throw her head back and laugh that big heartfelt guffaw. This challenge helped me develop a sharp fast sense of humor that serves me in so many ways. I love to make people laugh. The gift she bestowed on me by encouraging me to express myself creatively has served me continually and permitted me to shine.

When I was about seven years old, my mother asked me if I wanted to take ballet lessons or play the piano. I told her I wanted to play the guitar like Elvis Presley. The next thing I knew I was taking guitar lessons and was the proud owner of a small copper speckled electric guitar and a little amplifier. I was in heaven. I would sit and strum a G chord for hours.

Mom encouraged me to start my first band in grammar school (the Cracker and the Four Crumbs) and I played and sang at every family event for years. As I got older and branched out, she drove me or made my dad drive me to rock band rehearsals. She designed and sewed the best fake leopard bell-bottom pants ever for my first live rock gig. I still have the pants. I cannot bear to throw them away. Sadly, I'll never get in them again!

Ironically, as I got older and began to stake my claim in life and the road got rockier with my mom, my music saved me and protected me against the growing conflict. I could write and sing and pour out the big feelings. Art and creativity showed me a healthy path to recovery and self-worth and at that time, relief from the person who encouraged this expression.

All through high school and college she came to every coffee house show I would let her come to and she stood in the heat and pressing crowds at Folk Festivals and outdoor shows as my fame got a little bigger. After my college graduation, I insisted I move to New York to become rich and famous. She exploded and resisted. Yet even as she ranted, she always asked about my singing and how it was going.

After a few years of trying to become a star, I stopped performing and she was crushed. She asked me for years if I was ever going to sing again and I would get so annoyed and impatient when she did. Even when she was so sick toward the last days of her life, she told me I must start singing again. It hit me then and there that her belief in me and in "my talent" ran through our entire lives together. I made a promise to her that day that I would start singing and writing again.

All my life, when I write or create, I never face a blank page. The work may not be brilliant, but it always flows. I attribute this ease to my mother and her belief in me as an artist and her encouragement and awe of my process. After all, if your Mother lets you know that art and creativity are the things of grace and wonder and you are special for being creative, what more do you need?

The time I spent as my mother's caregiver watching dementia rob her of her proud spirit broke open my heart so it would safely heal back up. It was a time of forgiveness, understanding, and empathy. My mom was no longer my antagonist. She was no longer domineering. She was no longer telling me what to do or how to live. She was fighting for her own life, her strength now devoted to holding on to her dignity and pride.

The memories I have now of my mom are not of the arguments or screaming matches, but of the look of pride on her face on the side of the stage, the joy I see as she looks at me in old photos, and the holidays she celebrated with style and such enthusiasm.

I think it's time to get the guitar out from under the bed and sing a song in honor of my fiercest fan. And bless her dementia for bringing her back to me.

About the Author: Susanne White has over two decades of caregiving experience and has become a leading spokesperson and influencer for the caregiving community with her blog and website: caregiverwarrior.com. Susanne became a caregiver overnight when her father collapsed from exhaustion and heart issues, and her mother became disoriented and traumatized and diagnosed with dementia. Standing on the brink of caregiver burnout and panic, she began to come up with ways to manage her anxiety and fear of failure and ended up having the most profound and wonderful journey of her life. She shares the experience, strength, and hope she received caring for her parents and other family members so that she can help other caregivers care for themselves as they care for others.

Follow her on Twitter @caregivewarrior, Facebook, and Instagram @caregiverwarrior.

A Simple, Complex Man
Marianne Sciucco

Fred was diagnosed with mixed dementia in 2016 at the age of 79 and passed away in 2018. He was 81.

Who is this man my mom is hanging around with? I asked when he kept showing up at the house.

Widowed six years, Mom never showed any inclinations toward dating, a second marriage, or a new husband. Raising four kids on her own and working a full-time job left little time for a social life. But suddenly she had a boyfriend.

She said she felt awkward attending church dances and social functions with her friends and their husbands, dateless. She wanted someone to dance with, someone she didn't have to share. So, Fred came into our lives. He wined and dined her both at expensive restaurants and his home, showered her with gifts, luxuries she would not have indulged in on her own. The perfect boyfriend. At 55, she was captivated.

Our home was open to a steady stream of visitors, family, and friends, a gathering place where all of us entertained freely. We threw lots of impromptu parties, and last-minute dinner guests and sleepovers were the norm. Fred joined right in, becoming a permanent fixture. He and Mom dated five years before tying the knot. She was 60. He was 51. Their marriage lasted 30 years.

My stepfather was both a simple and a complex man. A premature infant born in 1936, he suffered a brain injury that impacted his cognitive abilities and left him with a speech impediment. The last of four sons born to a well-to-do family of professionals - businessmen, lawyers, and doctors - he didn't quite fit in. As a boy his parents coddled and protected him. As a teen he spent years in a residential school for children with mental impairments. He had rudimentary skills, could not read or write, or perform simple math. My mother accepted these deficits. She always looked for the best in others and possessed a forgiving nature, attributes she'd need to rely on heavily throughout their years together.

Fred's mother was the foundation of his world. After the death of his father, he lived with her until she passed away. The two traveled the country and the world and he spoke of these experiences as some of the best in his life. He depended on her to attend to their basic needs and did not need to function as an adult until after she died. In his mid-forties, he had to learn to manage bank accounts and monthly bills. With the help of tellers at his bank he fashioned a system that kept him on top of his personal business, never falling behind in his obligations, and was rightly proud of this.

He worked 30 years full-time as an aide in the kitchen of a VA hospital, rising at 5:00 AM to make it to work on time at 5:30. He washed pots and pans and mopped floors until the afternoon. Co-workers bullied and harassed him because of his speech impediment and low IQ. He hated it. Many times, he'd quit that job, but Mom always made him go back to rescind his notice because he was *so close* to his pension. He finally completed his term of service and retired to enjoy the benefits of his lifelong labor.

In many ways, Fred was childlike, and this impacted his relationships with my mother's children and those she loved. Possessive and jealous, he instigated big blowouts with just about all of us that would result in periods of estrangement which troubled my mother deeply. She simply wanted everyone to get along and did not understand that her husband's words and actions were intolerable and unacceptable. "You have to put up with him," I once told her. "We do not."

She chose her husband. He provided her with financial stability and a lovely home. They were happy together. He could have done without any of us. She could not, and because we loved her, we didn't stay away for long, perpetuating the cycle. For years there would be blowouts followed by estrangements and then making up, cardinal signs of a dysfunctional relationship. This went on for decades.

During some of our arguments I'd warn him: "You'd better be nice to me. I'm the one who will pick out your nursing home." He'd laugh at me and say, "I'm not going to a nursing home."

In November 2015, I went to visit Mom. I lived 250 miles away and faithfully made the trip each month. When I walked into the house and saw Fred, I didn't recognize him. Disheveled, unbathed, and unshaven, he looked like he hadn't had a haircut in months, and his clothes were tattered and dirty. This was so unlike the man who always took pride in his appearance, was well-groomed, and wore fine clothing.

"What's going on?" I asked my mother right after we said hello. He sat at the kitchen table silently, no greeting, as though I wasn't there.

"I don't know what to do with him anymore," she said. "Can you help me?"

He had been sliding downhill for months, exhibiting bizarre and inappropriate behaviors, repeating nonsensical monologues, picking fights with visitors, insulting and offending them. He possessed a talent for uncovering a person's deepest pain and regret and attacked it with cruelty, causing great emotional harm. Friends and family called me to report on these altercations and I experienced them myself on my own visits. Mom, hard of hearing, missed half of it and couldn't understand why people would get upset and leave. He spent the best part of each day sleeping in his recliner, woke only for meals, and then stayed up late into the night eating ice cream and junk food, talking nonsense to himself. This alteration in his personal appearance demonstrated one more example of a change in his cognition, one that could not be simply explained as, "He's just being Fred." Intervention could not be avoided.

I arranged for him to see a geriatric specialist. At the first visit, she took me aside and gave me the diagnosis: dementia. I was left to explain this to him and my mother who, deep in denial, refused to believe. I took him for an MRI of his brain which showed evidence of long-term trauma. He underwent neurological and psychiatric workups, both of which I witnessed, my heart sinking as his mental decline could not be denied. Throughout all of this Mom's health had also begun to deteriorate and she could not attend these consultations. *How would I tell her the results of these examinations?* I worried on the ride home, as he sat silently in the passenger seat, oblivious to what had just happened and the changes that were about to be imposed on his life.

He then spent five weeks in a hospital for geriatric psychiatry. The doctors diagnosed him with mixed dementia: frontotemporal, vascular, and Alzheimer's. He needed to be placed in a memory care unit immediately for his own safety and that of others. During his hospital stay he became violent, hitting, kicking, and pinching the staff. By now my mother's condition made it impossible for her to manage him at home. I found a facility 10 minutes from their home and he lived there 18 months until he peacefully passed away at age 81.

As I said, Fred was both a simple and a complex man. Born with brain damage he managed to live a productive and rewarding life and experienced much happiness and more good times than most people do. He was a hard worker, a devoted son and husband, a disrupter and a lover, and a jokester and a prank artist who loved to laugh and make others laugh. He didn't have a care in the world, paid no attention to current events, and lived for the moment. He had nerves of steel and a steady resolve. He stopped drinking when my mother said she wouldn't marry him if he didn't. He never took another drink. He smoked for decades and quit cold turkey. He got a driver's license in his fifties and bought himself a car. He drove until dementia made him dangerous on the road and willingly gave it up.

When I think of him now, I think of him in the pre-dementia days, when we spent time together at the beach, or sat at the kitchen table drinking coffee and talking, or enjoyed the delicious lobster dinners he brought, and the parties we threw at his house where we'd dance the night away to 80's alternative rock.

When I think of him now, I'm filled with sadness for the way his life ended. His confusion. His behavior problems that led to a terrible diagnosis and eventually removed him from his home. The fear he must have felt in the hospital as he begged us to take him home. "I'll be good," he cried. "I'm not sick." His fury at being locked into a dementia ward. The haze of the psychotropic drugs administered to control his violent behaviors, that turned him into a zombie. I am haunted by my role in all of this, a role I did not relish but assumed in the best interests of my mother. I upheld my promises to her as best as I could and helped make her final years comfortable. But it came at a great cost to all of us. Dementia is a horrible disease and breaks everyone involved in one way or another.

About the Author: Marianne Sciucco is not a nurse who writes but a writer who happens to be a nurse, using her skills and experience to create stories that bear witness to the humanity in all of us. She writes contemporary, women's, and young adult fiction.

A lover of words and books, she studied the craft of writing as an English major at the University of Massachusetts at Boston and worked for a time as a newspaper reporter in New England. She eventually became a registered nurse to avoid poverty.

With more than 20-years experience as a staff nurse and case manager, she's worked with countless families dealing with issues related to aging, elder care, Alzheimer's, and nursing home placement. In 2002, she put the two together and began writing about the intricate lives of people struggling with health and family issues. She published her debut novel, *Blue Hydrangeas, an Alzheimer's love story,* in 2013 to glowing reviews.

This book led her to become a co-founder and director of AlzAuthors, the global community of authors writing about Alzheimer's and dementia from personal experience to light the way for others. Visit AlzAuthors.com.

Marianne has written an award-winning prequel to *Blue Hydrangeas* called *Christmas at Blue Hydrangeas* and is currently working on *A Wedding at Blue Hydrangeas.* She is the author of *Swim Season,* a young adult novel based on her 11-years' experience as a Swim Mom in club, high school, and collegiate swimming.

She has also written several short stories, including *Ino's Love, Collection*, and *Birthday Party*.

All of her work is available in Kindle, audiobook, and paperback.

When not writing she works as a campus nurse at a community college in New York's Hudson Valley.

Follow Marianne on her blog MarianneSciucco.com, Twitter, Facebook, and LinkedIn.

The Last Dance
Phyllis Joly Greenberg

Evelyn Roseanna Joly (nee Boisvert) was born March 28, 1923. She passed away on May 10, 2002, at the age of 79. Evelyn and three of her sisters were diagnosed with Alzheimer's disease by the age of 72, including Louise Simmons, Lucille Sentener, and Claire Giordano. One of her four brothers, Larry Boisvert, was diagnosed with Alzheimer's in his mid-80s. Their father had Alzheimer's disease, though it was called "hardening of the arteries" when he died in 1966 at the age of 77.

My mother was the sixth of 10 children, born in a Connecticut mill town. My grandparents, French Canadians, became citizens in December 1946. All of their children were born in the United States. They lived in factory housing.

Evelyn lived within three miles of her birthplace most of her life, staying connected to sisters, brothers, and friends. She quit high school to work in the American Thread Company. It was the Depression. Recently, we found a leather notebook from her high school science class. In beautiful handwriting, the notes were detailed with diagrams and drawings labeled and shaded with colored pencils. It was obvious that she loved school. Folded inside were some report cards from grammar school and a pamphlet from a radio program with phrases to improve her French speaking skills. Many years later, both she and my dad took classes and earned their GED, not because they needed to but because they wanted to.

Evelyn Boisvert met my father, Alphonse Joly, at the French Club where he played the fiddle in his best friend's band. They were 17 when they had their first dance. Al took the bus 15 miles to see his gal. They were married at St. Mary's Church in 1942, three months before he joined the Navy. They were 19 years old. She was able to join him in Key West, FL after the invasion of Normandy when his ship was recommissioned for the war in the Pacific. She took a train south where my dad found her a little cottage near other navy wives. I am a result of that six-month reunion, born in 1945. Completing a family of five were my sister Linda in '48 and my brother David in '53.

When Dad was discharged after the war we lived in a basement apartment until they bought an old country house about a mile from town. The house was on a busy country road and Mom was afraid when my father worked the second shift. She was accustomed to living closer to neighbors.

My father was the dreamer. My mother was the practical thinker. In 1955 my mother heard from a friend about a tract of houses being built; all the same model on "Circle Drive." She convinced my dad that the old house had a coal-burning furnace, windows, and insulation needing to be replaced. The new ranch-style house was 920 square feet with a basement, wood floors, and baseboard heating in each room. It would be easier to maintain. She said that if they bought an "automatic washer" to replace the wringer washing machine she would get a part-time job.

True to her word, my mom found a factory job from 5:00-10:00 PM. By then, my dad was working days. She'd put a chicken in the oven or a pot of stew on the stove and my dad would complete the meal. Indeed, they shared the work in and out of the home. At first, she was the only working mother in the neighborhood and the family. I still remember the smell of Jean Nate as she prepared to leave for work, sometimes on a hot and humid summer day. She worked there for eight years.

Eventually, my mother started a small daycare in the house for up to three children. There were lots of kids in the neighborhood and some of the mothers were finding work. There was a backyard for them to play in and toys in a box. She overheard one of the kids tell a new kid not to do something. He said, "When Mrs. Joly says something, she means it." Right out of the mouth of babes. One day this same boy was having so much fun that he cried when his mother picked him up saying, "I want to be a Joly Boy." She took pride in caring for these children knowing their need for love, attention, and boundaries.

Our house was seven miles from the University. After I finished college, my mother found a job as a kitchen assistant in an independent dorm with 66 students. She left the house, rain or snow, at 5:00 AM Monday-Friday where she alone prepared the breakfast. The cook came in mid-morning and my mother left after lunch. When he left for another job she heard about two applicants and had reliable information that one of them took home expensive cuts of meat. She told the supervisor that she would leave her position if this cook was hired. They hired the other applicant and she had several more good years working there.

Evelyn was a person of principle. She was not a pushover either. One morning she walked into the dining room to find food thrown over the walls, floor, and tables, about the time *Animal House* was in the theaters. She locked the door to the kitchen and didn't put out the buffet of cereals, juices, and breads. No made-to-order eggs, bacon, sausage, and home fries would be available until the dining room was clean. The first students to arrive claimed to not be responsible for the mess. When that didn't impress "Evie," as they called her, they gathered others to clean up. She provided the buckets and cleaning materials until it met her standards of cleanliness. Recently we found a yellow and white gingham apron with the name "Evie" across the front given to her by the students.

Retirement in the '80s offered my parents the luxury of time to do more traveling in their RV which also served as a portable home to spend winters in Florida. Retirement found them busier than ever! My mother made quilts for each of us and the grandchildren. They took square dancing lessons. My dad joined a local band that played at nursing homes and other community events. My mother usually went along for the camaraderie tapping her foot to the music. She especially loved the old French-Canadian songs.

Evelyn loved her nights out for bingo. When I would visit in the summer she suggested that she didn't need to go. I assured her that my visit should not interrupt her weekly bingo night. In the years when she was showing significant problems with short-term memory, I went to bingo with her. She had five cards and didn't miss a beat and then inspected my two cards, finding some missed spots. Amazing.

We led a simple life by today's standards but our parents provided everything that we needed. We lived in a small but clean house and had three home-cooked meals a day by which you could set the clock. When we got home from school we would find Mom ironing (remember those days) while watching the *Art Linkletter's House Party*. Our clothes were not extravagant but we always had the appropriate clothing for school, church, and play. Everyone had a chore. And we didn't try to do anything behind our mom's back because she would know.

Mom met the Gold Standard. She was not our playmate. Instead, she was our conscience, teacher, and someone who we knew would fight to keep us safe. She taught us that pride was in the doing not in the bragging. In her quiet way, she was our best cheerleader by setting a standard for respect for ourselves and others.

On May 10, 2002, my Dad was playing his fiddle in his band at a Mother's Day luncheon for the Seniors Club. My mother was sitting with friends and called him over saying that she wanted to dance. He put down his fiddle and they waltzed to a slow song. As he was returning to the band Mom collapsed. She died that day at the hospital. It started with a dance and ended with a dance; 59 ½ years of commitment, love, and grace.

About the Author: Phyllis Joly Greenberg is retired and living in California. She worked in public schools as a teacher, counselor, and school psychologist. She was married to Morris Greenberg for 43 years. She was his caregiver as his condition declined from Lewy body dementia. The story Phyllis wrote about Morris, "East to West: The Making of a Family" is in *Before the Diagnosis: Stories of Life and Love Before Dementia.*

Cheese Rolls and a Punnet of Plums
Deb Bunt

Suffolk born Peter Berry was diagnosed with early-onset dementia at the age of 50. Now 56, Peter spends his time cycling and raising awareness about the condition. He has raised £20,000 for dementia charities through his two cycling challenges, one of which was done on a penny farthing bike. Peter continues to live well with dementia and, on average, cycles between 800 – 1,000 miles a month. After years of trying, Peter has finally converted his wife, Teresa, to the joys of cycling and the couple have now cycled many hundreds of miles together.

One summer's day in 1981, a fresh-faced seventeen-year-old Peter Berry told his father he was going to cycle the eighty-mile journey to Cromer[1]. When his father, Jimmy, asked him if he knew the way, Peter assured him that he could get certainly get himself to Lowestoft[2].

Ever pragmatic and never one to panic, Jimmy said, "Well, keep the sea on your right, boy, keep pedalling and you'll soon find Cromer."

Peter has never forgotten those words or the excitement of setting off early one morning on his four-speed bike, wearing shorts and a tee-shirt and fuelled by Mars bars, chewing gum, and two cheese rolls.

By lunchtime, the young Peter had arrived in Cromer, eaten the cheese rolls, bought some fish and chips, and was sitting on a bench above the beach, surveying the scene below.

"I sat there," he recalled, "and then I didn't really know what to do. My plan had been to stay the night somewhere and cycle home the next day. I put some gum in my mouth and looked at everyone around me. Then I came to realise that Cromer was full of old people. I got bored very quickly. So, I stuck the gum under the bench - I know, what a young hoodlum I was - and cycled home. I got home at about ten o'clock. All Father said was, 'did you have a good time, Peter, my boy?' And I suppose I did! But I was already plotting the next adventure so I thought no more of it."

Until recently, that is. For the last few months, Peter has talked a great deal about this trip and its importance. Although he couldn't say exactly what it represented to him, he talked of an increasing compulsion to retrace that one-hundred-and-sixty-mile round trip.

There followed a few weeks of planning and much anticipatory pleasure in putting "project Cromer" into action. The night before we set out, Peter sent me one of his messages, conceived in his foggy and tired mind, but bursting into my world as a perfectly formed image: "My thoughts are like sand through my fingers. My only hope is that they are saved by others and panned as if looking for gold, the precious metals that are my memories."

On June 16th on quite possibly the hottest day of the year and a bit more sedately (and with neither Mars bars nor cheese rolls to weigh us down), a quirky quartet of cyclists left Suffolk to accompany Peter in panning for some of these old, precious memories.

The four comprised: Peter (choosing to cycle this distance on his single speed bike, "just to make it a challenge," he said), Teresa, his wife (now a fully converted cyclist with a wardrobe full of cycling clothes, enough to make Imelda Marcos concede defeat in a face-off between shoes and lycra), Peter's old school friend, Mark (still sporting an impressive array of injuries from various accidents) and me (fuelled by a Peter-driven enthusiasm and his zest for life).

With the sun beating down on us, we cycled through the familiar Suffolk countryside and soon reached Norfolk. Every now and again, some landscape or a building would trigger Peter's memory, bringing forth joyous exclamations.

"The golf course!" he announced at one point. "I thought it was here. And 'round the corner, there should be a pub. I stopped here for a drink of lemonade. I engraved my initials into the outside of the pub wall so there would always be a bit of me in Norfolk!"

And whilst there certainly was a golf course, there was, alas, no pub. It had been demolished and the area was now sealed off. All that remained was a pile of rubble, strewn haphazardly over the yellowing grass and the jagged remnants of broken bottles.

"Well, that's scuppered my attempts to write my initials again," said Peter, and I thought I could hear just a touch of sorrow in his voice for the loss of the pub, the wall, and, more importantly, for the loss of the tangible evidence of him ever having been there.

We reached Cromer by late afternoon in various states of physical and sartorial disarray. The sunshine had been unremitting; there are, undoubtedly, many things which are less pleasant in life than damp, sweaty lycra clinging to damp sweaty bodies but at that moment, neither Mark, Teresa, nor I were able to articulate what these things might be. Needless to say, the only one in our little party who looked fresh and energised was Peter. Peter was living proof of his doctrine: "If I keep the bit below my eyebrows healthy, then it should help the bit above my eyebrows." Here he was: the personification of that maxim, barely out of breath and singularly unruffled by the miles which he had pedalled.

The next day heralded Peter's seminal moment. We made our way to the beach and climbed up the concrete steps until we were high above the sea and the promenade. Peter found the bench he had sat on all those years ago. The chip shop he had recalled with such fondness was now an Indian take-away but there were many other parts of Cromer which Peter remembered well.

We huddled around Peter, as if forming an impenetrable barrier to keep intruders from disturbing him, whilst he sat on the bench, side-by-side with his private reverie. We could see the figures below, like a scene from a Bruegel painting: a mass of people, scurrying around busily, searching for something, although who knew what? Perhaps they were hunting for their future selves? Maybe they were trying to recreate the past. Perhaps I am just being fanciful, as is my wont, caught up in Peter's whimsical moment.

This was a trip Peter had been anticipating for many months; something he had talked about consistently, something which was fundamental to his very core. And now, here we were. I wondered what the emotional impact might be on Peter, whether he had been transported back to the past and, if he had, what that was like for him, armed as he was now with the knowledge of his future self.

As Peter looked around at the scene playing itself out below, he said, "Here's a thing. Forty years ago, I thought Cromer was full of old people; today, we are the old people."

We laughed but he was right; like it or not, aging is something which comes to us all whilst we live, only to stop when we die. We were, indeed, the next generation to be shunted along on the clunking conveyer belt of life.

A surreptitious grope under the bench for Peter yielded an interesting discovery: a small, crusty, but well-compacted mound of gum was still attached to the bench. It's hard to say with any certainty if it was the same gum Peter had deposited all those years ago but, curiously, no one was prepared to taste it or to bring it back to Suffolk for a more scientific exploration of its composition.

You know, I think we were all moved in our own ways about accompanying Peter on his journey to meet the seventeen-year-old callow youth. Mark summed it up when he said to Peter: "Thank you for letting us be part of your old and new memories."

But in hindsight, I don't think I had really appreciated what an emotional journey this had been for Peter. When we were back in Suffolk and talking through our adventure he said, "Here's a thing, Deb. I sat on that bench next to the young me. How many people get a chance to do something like that? I recreated something from forty years ago. And, you know, I looked at the young me and I felt quite moved."

"What would you have said to the young you?" I asked. As always with Peter, I was curious to know how he processed events.

"I would have looked him in the eye and told him that the future would be ok; yes, despite everything, I would have told that young lad that the future would be absolutely fine."

He gave me one of his showman beams, a smile that stretches right across his face. It's a smile that seems to mask all melancholy unless you look closely into Peter's eyes. Only then, when you have pierced through the film of the showman front and the film crinkles and disintegrates under the pressure, you might see the occasional flicker of sadness.

"You know, this trip was important. It was so much more than a cycling trip. I was able to harvest a moment from the past and that's so important as I can't sow the seeds for the future."

As ever, Peter's perspective on life and his determination that his glass will remain half-full created conflicting emotions within me. I continue to admire his combative attitude to the ever-encroaching dementia, his fist waving defiance, and I wish I had half of his iron will. I know I still allow myself to get entangled in the meaningless mesh of life's trivialities.

This got me to thinking: when I was a small child, my parents, keen Gilbert and Sullivan fans, used to sing to me and these lines sprung to my mind:

"Life's a pudding full of plum
care's a canker that benumbs;
wherefore waste our elocution,
on impossible solution?
Life's a pleasant institution,
let us take it as it comes…
…String the lyre and fill the cup,
lest on sorrow we should sup."[3]

Peter is the perfect embodiment of Gilbert's words: he takes each day, each hour, each minute, each moment as it comes. His cup is as full as he can make it. Life may well be a "pudding full of plums," but discerning grocer that he has become, Peter extracts each sweet plum from the punnet and feasts on it with epicurean pleasure. If any rancid plums make it to his mouth, he spits them out.

Although Peter's outlook on life is something which I intellectually understand, I am still emotionally not always able to put his teaching into action. I still experience angst about trivial things. I worry about the future and stress about things over which I have no control. Oh, I know I have a long way to travel (almost definitely beyond Cromer!) before I reach Peter's state of mind.

Paradoxically it appears that it takes a man with dementia to teach a woman without dementia how to live well, how to appreciate life, and quite simply, how "to take life as it comes."

[1] Cromer is a seaside town in Norfolk, England.
[2] Lowestoft is a seaside town in Suffolk County, England, and the two East Anglian counties sit next to each other.
[3] Taken from *The Gondoliers* by WS Gilbert and AS Sullivan.

About the Author: Deb Bunt moved to Suffolk in 2018 and she and Peter became close friends and cycling buddies. Deb spent six years in New York, working at the United Nations, before returning to the UK where she worked as a parenting practitioner in London. Her main ambition in life had always been to be a writer and so, when she met Peter, she was able to fulfill this ambition by writing Peter's book *Slow Puncture, Living Well with Dementia*. Deb is married to Martin, has two grown up sons, one grandson, one granddaughter, and spends her days cycling, writing, promoting Peter's activities and, as Peter's late father would have said, "learning all the time." You can find her on Facebook, Twitter and LinkedIn.

You can also connect with Peter Berry on Facebook and Twitter or on his website https://peterberrylwa.wixsite.com/peterberry.

Toodie's Story
Grant Hill

Ann Hill was evaluated with cognitive impairment in 2015. As her symptoms progressed, she received a more definitive diagnosis of Lewy body dementia in 2018. Her speech and cognitive abilities diminished to the point that she needed constant care. She resided with her husband and son who were her primary caregivers during the pandemic until she passed away in February 2022.

The following four essays are about Ann Hill, written by people who loved her. This first essay is written by her husband.

Ann was born and raised in Long Beach in a large Irish Catholic family and, being the youngest, was everyone's favorite. She went to the neighborhood church for grammar school, the same church where her parents were wed, and the one we were married in years later. Her family gave her the nickname Toodie, when she was very young, a name her old friends and family still call her. She attended Poly High School and completed her college studies and education at San Diego State. We are very grateful for her lifelong friendships that have continued today.

Her mother, after raising eight kids, worked for the Long Beach Unified School District. Many of their close family friends were longtime administrators and teachers in the district. It was natural for Ann to follow in those footsteps; her love, support, kindness, and guidance of young children was her passion. Her friends, parents, principals, and colleagues took notice and would place those kids who needed that loving touch with Ann. In her over thirty years with the school district, Ann taught kindergarten, first, and second grade.

Ann started her first few years of teaching at Birney Elementary School, where many other young teachers were also starting their careers. They bonded, worked, and helped each other figure out this teaching thing, sharing supplies, doing lesson plans, and trading ideas. There were more experienced teachers helping the newbies along, and many of them are still friends. I really enjoyed helping her in the classroom, grading papers, preparing the many projects, putting up bulletin boards, and trying to make the classroom her own.

Each school year Ann would take pictures of all her students at the beginning of the year, during holidays, at events, and on class trips. By the end of the year, we had hundreds of printed pictures. Near the end of the school year, we would make unique scrapbooks for each student to give to their parents. We would spend weeks applying Ann's Creative Memories touches to these books to make them special for each family. We still have shoeboxes filled with pictures of her students from all the past years.

Occasionally, I would try and talk my way into some of her fun field trips. Who doesn't like the zoo? She had many families, with multiple siblings, whose parents would insist Mrs. Hill be their child's teacher and there were always plenty of parents volunteering in her class.

We were married in 1986, and during these working years tried unsuccessfully to have our own children, enduring numerous reproductive procedures. Finally, we were blessed with the arrival of Connor, our only child. After two years of staying at home, Ann went back to the classroom, this time to Twain Elementary. There she met and worked with some wonderful teachers and new lifelong friends. Ann was always caring and thinking of others and there was not a birthday she would forget. She would recognize every student's birthday who came through her classroom. Her memory of every family member's birthday, for both her family and mine, was mind-boggling. There was always a card to send, a gift to wrap or a party to attend. In return, her classroom families recognized her during the holidays and special occasions. I still remember the many years we got these fantastic Christmas tamales from one family who had four children go through Ann's class.

Our family of three loved to get outdoors as much as possible. Ann and I followed Connor's activities: Cub Scouts, Little League, soccer teams, and sailing classes. She loved being a team mom! Whether it was road trip vacations to the Northwest, cruises to Mexico, camping trips or just going to the beach, Ann planned and organized these adventures to the extreme. I would do the heavy lifting, but she was in charge, provided I did the driving.

I have been a sailor for most of my life, and when we were first dating, I would take Ann out sailing in my racing dinghy. We eventually did some boat races and of course, you are bound to get wet and cold. It wasn't until after we got married, she told me she hated that small boat stuff. She would say, "You go out and have fun, I'll come down for the party." Ann did like sailing to Catalina, in my family's larger sailboat, during the summer.

Ann always wanted to travel more, and we talked about going to Ireland, Europe, the East Coast, and other exotic worlds. But life got in the way, and when her condition made her stop teaching, I realized her time to travel was getting limited. We planned a two-week trip to the East Coast, visiting Washington DC and New York City. The plane trip went okay, but going through the airport and the TSA scanner, she was easily confused by their instructions. We saw the great monuments of our Nation's Capital, took tours of the Big Apple, the Empire State Building, museums, the Statue of Liberty, and a play on Broadway. Ann was happy and we both enjoyed this great adventure. She was able to do all the walking and tours, but I was always concerned I would lose her. So, each morning, I would dress her in a jacket, and place her cell phone in a buttoned pocket. The phone had a location app, and I could see on my phone where she was. It did come in handy a few times.

The following year, our son Connor, graduated from Cal State Long Beach, and we were fortunate that her condition allowed her to be the proud parent, looking on. We feel our parenting raised a pretty good kid and Ann's kindness to others has been passed on.

Connor and I have these wonderful memories and think somewhere deep in Ann's memory, the images, thoughts, experiences, and happiness are still buried deep within her. I believe there will be a time when both of our minds will be back together so we can share these times.

About the Author: Grant Hill, also from Long Beach, grew up in a family of teachers. After receiving an engineering degree from Long Beach State, he had a 35-year aerospace career with the Boeing Company. The three of them reside in Cypress, where "two clumsy guys are taking care of mom."

Toodie, The Early Years
Teri Hayes McGuire

This second essay about Ann Hill is written by her older sister.

My name is Teri and I am one of Ann's older sisters. I was the closest in age being four years older.

There were eight children in our family beginning with Paul, Mick, Penny, Jim, Joanne, myself, Joe, and Ann. There was an 11-year period from start to finish so as you can imagine, she was born into a very lively household.

Ann was a premature baby at 5 pounds 8 ounces. It seemed she had a hard time thriving and was a rather frail baby, but my mom had lots of willing helpers to pitch in and care for her. She would forever be the youngest and last child. We were all protective of her, a feeling I still carry.

My dad was a jokester and was quick to give you a nickname. I am often asked where the name Toodie came from. The short story is it came from one of the first words uttered by my baby sister. We would gather as a family and watch TV at night. It was the early sixties and there was a favorite show called *Car 54, Where Are You?* and on it, there was a police officer named Tutti. For whatever reason Ann would say the name Tutti, I want to watch Tutti. The name stuck, and the spelling adjusted and "Toodie" had her nickname. Other nicknames followed but none stuck like Toodie and until this day it's what family members and childhood friends still call her.

There would be more nicknames mostly associated with her slight build and lack of interest in food. She was "The Bird" and Twiggy. I think you could count maybe five foods she liked. Kraft Mac and Cheese was one, and her birthday meal, cream chipped beef on crackers. Don't ask me why but she loved it!

We lived in a neighborhood full of large Catholic families. Maybe not as large as ours but there were lots of kids to play with whatever age you were. There was always a game of hide-and-seek going on or a ball game in the street. Being the youngest was hard in this situation and being of slight build didn't help either. Poor Toodie would get in the way, which resulted in many accidents. The worst one was when my sister Penny swung a bat back and hit Toodie in the eye. It was the worst day. Penny felt horrible and our baby girl had one hell of a goose egg. Fortunately, there was no permanent damage but the eye took a while to heal and we all watched the colors change on her face.

Being from such a large family the girls shared a bedroom. We had two sets of bunkbeds with the younger girls having the bottom bunks. There were many nights when we would end up sleeping together from a bad dream or being cold. One night we were all having trouble sleeping, excited because we were leaving on our summer vacation the next day. For many years we would rent a cabin in Twin Peaks in our local mountains for a week. Toodie ended up in bed with me that night and for some reason (not on purpose) I pushed her out of bed. It was not much of a drop from the bed to the floor, but she ended up breaking her arm. None of the kids believed she was badly hurt because we didn't want a delay to our beloved mountains, but Mom insisted on taking her to the hospital. They didn't see anything broken on the x-ray, so with her arm in a sling, we were off without too much delay. She was still in pain and by the next day there was another trip to the hospital. This x-ray revealed that there was a break. It was an especially tough vacation for her and me. She was miserable and I felt terrible and to this day it's always bothered me. It didn't help over the years when sharing family stories that everyone remembers when Teri pushed Toodie out of bed.

In a large family there is a lot of teasing going on, and ours was no exception. Toodie and Joe, the youngest, were arch enemies. They were at each other constantly. Joe was relentless but Toodie was cunning. We were playing hide and seek in the house one night when Mom and Dad were out. Joe had hidden in the dryer and Toodie knew he was in there. I was closely watching this play out. Toodie went to the dryer and with a look of "I got ya", pressed the button on the dryer and Joe went tumbling! He escaped with no damage but to his ego. When Mom and Dad got home that night, Joe ran to the car and yelled "Toodie turned me on!" Good one Toodie!

We were very lucky to have kids in our neighborhood of our own age to play with. Toodie had Jamie and Annie. She was friends with both for many years. Loyalty is one of her strongest virtues which Ann carried into adulthood. She never forgot a birthday and often sent holiday cards as well. She took time for people. As a sister, she was very loyal to me. I was more of a wild child and believe me, she gave me grief about it, but I was still her sister and I always knew she was in my corner.

Being the youngest, Ann had a very special relationship with my parents. The nest was getting smaller each year until she was the only one left. They had a very special bond. She worked hard in school and became a wonderful teacher, wife, and mother. Our parents were so proud of her and were there for her every step and she for them. Losing them was hard for all of us but devastating for her. Ann was sensitive and carried her feelings on her sleeve. That's who she was, she cared deeply.

I remember when things started to change. I would get calls from Ann for years and there seemed to me many health issues, horrible painful problems with her feet, and bad headaches. Lots of doctor appointments. I heard the fear in her voice and it broke my heart. The reality of the diagnosis was hard to face. I remember my sister Joanne and I went over to visit Ann and Grant. She was holding a picture of my parents and stroking it lovingly. She looked at us both and told us, "this is my Mom and Dad." She didn't know us.

I'm so grateful Ann has Grant and Connor to love and care for her. I pray for them all daily and know when the time comes, Mom and Dad, and even Joe, our brother who passed away, will be waiting with loving arms on the other side.

About the Author: Teri McGuire is one of Ann's sisters. She grew up in Long Beach then moved to Palm Desert, California in her late twenties. She has worked in the travel industry for 35 years. Teri is married with three beautiful stepdaughters and three adorable grandchildren.

A Woman of Beauty
Mary Nelson

This third essay about Ann Hill is written by a dear friend.

I met Ann Hill on my first day at a new school in 1990. I was quite nervous because I had never taught 1st grade and found that Ann was going to be one of my grade level partners. She put me at ease right away and offered to help in any way she could. I was immediately impressed with her spirit of generosity and her professionalism. I was so comfortable, in fact, I told her I was newly pregnant with my first child. I later found out that Ann and her husband, Grant, had been trying to have a baby for several years.

Ann turned out to be a great friend! True to her word she helped guide me through the new grade and offered assistance many times! Thinking back, it must have been so difficult to see the teacher down the hall getting more and more pregnant as the school year went by, but Ann was always kind and considerate. She even planned my baby shower at school several months later.

Ann was a wonderful teacher and the students flourished in her classroom. She was innovative, worked hard, and provided a warm environment for the youngsters. There was a lot of learning and a lot of fun going on. Her love of children was evident in all that she did for her students!

Ann was as beautiful outside as she was inside. She was a stylish dresser with matching shoes and bags and was quite a fashion icon at the school. Her bright blond hair was lovely and her nails were always colorful and shiny. Although Ann seemed to have it all, I knew there was always that longing for her own child!

Several years later, after many medical interventions and a lot of personal anguish, Ann and Grant were finally going to have a baby. The teachers at school were thrilled for them and Ann actually glowed! Everything was perfect until a problem occurred and Ann had to spend the majority of her pregnancy in bed. Happily, the end result was the birth of her precious baby boy Connor!

I never again worked with Ann because she was able to stay home for a couple of years and be a mom. I know it was an amazingly happy time for her with her much-adored son. It was such great news when Ann was later placed at a different school where two of my very best friends also taught.

Ann and I have remained friends for over thirty years. I look back on the days we worked together with great fondness and many happy memories. When I see her today, I always remember the young woman thrilled to be having a baby at long last!

About the Author: Mary Nelson is a retired teacher from Long Beach, California. She is married and has two grown children. She loves hanging out with family and friends, traveling, reading, and being with her dogs!

Ann Hill, "Tuna Princess"
Donna Corn and Karla Lucas

This last essay about Ann Hill is written by two more dear friends.

It was in the spring of 1996 that we had the pleasure of meeting Ann Hill for the first time. She was planning to return to the classroom after being on a year-long maternity leave. At that time, Karla was considering returning from a job-sharing teaching position to a full-time position. Donna was looking to find a new partner with whom to share a teaching contract. The pieces all fell into place, and Ann joined the staff at Mark Twain Elementary School in the fall of 1996. We soon learned that not only did Ann bring a good deal of expertise into the classroom, but she also brought much laughter and friendship. She quickly endeared herself to students, families, and staff members alike.

We also discovered that Ann had a penchant for playing practical jokes, which we of course reciprocated. After being the recipients of many mischievous and playful jokes, we decided to go all out with an antic of our own.

Ann detested tuna of any kind, which made it hard to enjoy lunch with us, as we both would bring tuna regularly. She informed us that we could not bring tuna for lunch on the days that she was teaching. We decided to make advertisements for our school campus stating that Ann Hill was the new spokesperson for Chicken of the Sea tuna. Just for Ann, we created a personalized "Tuna Princess" parking spot, "Tuna Princess" business cards, and "Tuna Princess" posters all around the campus. All of them had a lovely picture of Ann in her newfound role. This antic on our part caused us to be the victims of many more practical shenanigans by Ann throughout our years together at Twain. She enlisted the help of our principal to pull off the ultimate retaliation, causing each of us in personalized situations to have momentary episodes of anxiety. We still laugh to this day about the fun times we had together with Ann.

As well as bringing us laughter and friendship, Ann brought thoughtfulness and generosity to our relationship. There was nothing she would not do for her friends. When Karla's husband passed away, Ann organized a collection of donations for the family from the school staff. When Donna's baby passed away, Ann organized a rose bush to be planted at the family's home with a remembrance plaque as a gift from the school staff. She had a tremendous heart for giving, and would typically bring us holiday treats, as well as just "thinking of you" surprises. Also, Ann loved to shop online. Being the stylish dresser that she was, she would often generously share her fashion finds with us.

Twenty-four years have passed since we first met Ann, and our lives have been enriched by her laughter, her friendship, and her generosity. Reflecting on these years brings us joy and love, as we remember our dear friend, and the vibrant spirit she brought to our lives. When we visit her now, we occasionally see a particular expression on her face, like a wink or a smile, and it brings us such vivid recollections of that spunky, fun-loving, sassy "Tuna Princess" Ann.

About the Authors: Donna and Karla have both retired from teaching. Donna is married, with three grown children, and lives in Garden Grove with her husband Clark. Karla is from Long Beach, with three grown children. Bonded by their many years of friendship, Donna and Karla spend time traveling and hanging out, enjoying their time together. Karla and Donna have been lifelong friends with Mary Nelson, with their friendships spanning over 50 years. Through Mary, Karla and Donna were introduced to Ann, who then became a teaching colleague, and more importantly, a dear friend.

Harmony
Renée Brown Harmon, MD

Harvey S. Harmon, MD was diagnosed with younger-onset Alzheimer's disease in 2010 at the age of 50. He passed away from complications of the disease in 2018.

I met Harvey in college. Actually, I can't say that I ever *met* Harvey. When you go to a small liberal arts college, you just know everyone, especially if you're in the same sciencey pre-med classes. He was a year ahead of me, but during one semester, we had three classes together, including French. I remember that he asked me to join him in a study session once, but I turned him down because I didn't *need* a study session. He later told me that he had admired me from afar for a while and especially liked my "springy ankles."

"My what?"

"I like the way you bounce when you walk!"

He didn't ask me out again until after he had graduated and I was a senior--to a Crosby, Stills & Nash concert. What I most remember about that first date was that he grabbed my hand and held on tight as we made our way through the throngs leaving the concert. He said that he didn't want to lose me in the crowd. We dated off and on after that, but it wasn't until he returned home from a six-week trip to Europe, called me, and we talked for hours on the phone that I realized that I *really* liked this guy. He was so kind. And gentle. And patient.

We dated in earnest and fell in love. When we were both accepted into the same medical school in the same year, that clinched it for us as a couple, and we were married the summer after our first year of med school. I'm not sure I could have made it through medical school without Harvey's gentle, quiet spirit keeping my stress in check. In the third year of medical school, Harvey and I both decided to pursue family medicine as a specialty, independent of each other, and for different reasons. We completed our residencies in Charleston, South Carolina, both of us selected as co-chief residents, then moved back to Birmingham, Alabama, our hometown, to practice medicine. These first seven years of marriage, medical school, and residency set the stage for our future life together. We were never competitive with each other, somehow managing to make the same grade point average, class rank and even board certification scores. We instinctively knew we were two halves of a whole, equals, and set out from the start to make our lives together reflect that mutual respect and equality, neither of us playing into the myth of gender roles.

It probably comes as no surprise that we wanted to practice together. It was our goal to share the responsibilities of a family medicine practice as well as share the responsibilities of raising a family and managing a household. When we started the practice, Double Oak Family Medicine, in 1992, I was pregnant with our first daughter. The practice was brand-new, and we were only seeing two to three patients a day, so it made sense that one of us would be at the office, and the other would be home with the baby. We alternated days at home and days at the practice, so that we were each part-time physicians. We eventually had two daughters, and as they grew, our practice did too, so that by the time they were in elementary school, the practice could support both of us being at the office until one of us left to pick up carpool, then stay with the girls the rest of the day. Our daughters had the advantage of being fully parented by both of us. Our patients and the staff readily accepted this arrangement as we were so similar in our approaches. The ultimate plan for the practice was for both of us to be full-time at the office when our youngest daughter turned sixteen and could drive herself.

Harvey had a little bit of a hard time knowing what to do with himself when he was outside of the office; he much preferred to be practicing medicine. He was a wonderful father, though. Reading aloud to the girls, playing basketball with them, or coaching their soccer teams, he was a constant presence in their lives. I treasure memories of him playing horse, one daughter on his back yelling for "Baldy," Harvey's horse name, to gallop faster. He enjoyed working in the yard, planting a small vegetable garden each year. And there was the line of family dogs: Miss Kyle, Blackie and Nash. Each dog knew to pick Harvey as his or her special person. They were *his* dogs. Running long distances eventually became his prime activity once the girls were in school.

Harvey was the consummate physician, even looking the part; tall and slender, with rimless glasses, button-down shirt, and tie, he always wore a long white lab coat, black stethoscope around his neck, pockets bulging with prescription pad and books. His patients loved him. He was kind, attentive, and patient, and the best listener I have ever known. He once called a three-year-old on the phone after he had removed a particularly painful splinter from her hand, just to make sure she wasn't mad at him. Another patient told me that he once emptied his brown paper lunch bag so that he could place some sample medications in it for her. I know of at least three patients that credit Harvey with saving their lives--and never tired of telling me so. It was as if he was born to be a physician.

***

Harvey was a marathon runner, and we, his family, his greatest fans. We attended most of his races, and armed with homemade signs and our loudest voices, we followed his progress by mapping out the course and strategically placing ourselves at points along the route. He was an amazing runner, and we were so proud of him!

Harvey always said that he was the best cross-country runner on his high school basketball team, but he didn't really take to running regularly until we were in medical school. He would say that running and training for 10Ks was his outlet for the mental and physical stress of medical school.

I'm not sure what tempted him to try his first marathon; maybe it was the challenge of it. We were back in Birmingham, with a new practice and a new baby. Was this life more stressful than the years of medical school and residency, and therefore, he needed longer time outdoors? In any event, he trained for his first marathon using training plans gleaned from the *Runner's World* magazine. He trained by himself in our neighborhood, and I remember helping him train for that first marathon by meeting him at preplanned points along his route with water, sports drinks and snacks. He would look miserable to me, salt encrusting his face, as he stretched his cramping leg muscles. At the end of that first marathon, he was pitiful; throwing up, shivering, barely able to walk, supported between his father and a friend. It took him three days to recover, as he limped around the office on punished legs. But the bug had bitten; he was hooked.

Harvey eventually was invited to join a running group who trained together for marathons. He had never run with others before, and this group quickly became his social circle. Harvey was inspired by this group, especially one member who had the nickname Hillmaster for his ability to sprint up the infamous hills in our area. This group of guys ran our area's yearly February marathon together, not as a pack, but individually, for about seven years. They even traveled to Chicago once to run the famed Chicago Marathon.

Eventually, Harvey surpassed even Hillmaster in speed and decided to train on his own. He kept perfecting his technique, trying different strides and training regimens that he had researched, all in an effort to remain injury-free and fast. He only ever suffered a few minor strains. I was always very proud of him, but would tease him about all the research he would do on running.

"Really, Harvey! What's there to learn? I'll teach you how to run. All you do is put one foot in front of the other over and over again, then do it faster and faster!"

Of course, he was in amazing physical shape, with a resting heart rate in the forties.

Harvey's marathon career took off when he started to train on his own. Not held back by the group, he could push himself to new limits. Yes, he was gone for a long time on training Saturdays, and would awake very early in the morning for weekday runs, but I never minded. We had learned to give each other space and time to develop our individual interests at this point in our marriage.

His times improved, and he eventually had a time that qualified him to run the Boston Marathon in 2009, a year before his Alzheimer's diagnosis. The Boston is run on a Monday, and we decided that he would go alone so that I could stay home and keep the practice open. All went well, and the office staff and I were able to track his progress because he was equipped with a computer chip that allowed us to watch his times. He did remarkably well. Another aspect of Harvey's running was his consistency. His interval mile times along the way were identical. He was a machine.

Boston was his last marathon before the diagnosis of Alzheimer's was made. He continued to run, of course, but now he had the luxury of time and could fully concentrate on improving his times. Harvey ran five more marathons after his diagnosis. He actually placed third in a small marathon in Jackson, Mississippi, and took home prize money. My husband was a professional athlete! He came in second in his age group in an Atlanta marathon. Harvey's personal best was in February 2011, just five months after he was diagnosed, with a time of three hours, thirteen minutes--a remarkable time for anyone at any age, but for someone with Alzheimer's disease? Amazing!

***

There was so much more to Harvey than his roles of husband, father, physician, and runner. I cannot fully explain how kind and patient he was. I called him my "rock" because he was always a steadying constant in our life together. He was never anxious or stressed, and he could calm my nerves with his unflappable demeanor or his gentle humor. When I beat myself up about some self-perceived fault—some missed opportunity or a failed attempt at something—his reply to me was, "Renée, you are a good person." This simple comment never failed to make me smile and bring me back to reality by pointing out the bigger picture and putting my supposed mistakes into perspective.

How I loved, and do still love, that man!

About the Author: Renée Brown Harmon, MD resides in Birmingham, Alabama, where she recently retired from a twenty-nine-year career in family medicine. She and her husband shared responsibilities at their medical practice and at home with two daughters until Alzheimer's disease forced his retirement. She is the author of *Surfing the Waves of Alzheimer's: Principles of Caregiving That Kept Me Upright*, portions of which appear in this essay. Her latest joy is becoming a grandmother to her first-born grandchild. You can connect with her on Facebook, Twitter and Instagram.

The Tie That Binds
LeAnn Morgan Miller and Jan Morgan Alexander

Linda Sue Raborn Morgan was diagnosed with Lewy body dementia in 2009. She passed away on August 16, 2011, at 70 years old.

As we are nearing the eleventh anniversary of our mom's death, we realize how much our family has changed. We miss her every day. She died after a four-year battle with Lewy body dementia.

Linda Sue Raborn was born March 5, 1941, in Lillie, Louisiana, to parents Aaron and Margaret Raborn. She had a younger brother, Bennie. They grew up in Springhill, Louisiana. She met her husband, Gerald Morgan, Jr., through a blind date set up by cousins. They married on August 6, 1960. They had three children: Keith, LeAnn, and Jan.

Our mom was the best mom ever. She raised us in church and taught us about Jesus. She and Dad went on most of our church trips. Glorieta, New Mexico, was her favorite. They took us tent camping every summer. We had some great adventures. Mom loved playing the piano. She really loved talking with her friends and boy could she talk! She always had long painted fingernails which we noticed as she pointed that finger at us to lecture. She and Dad loved playing cards with their friends. There were many rules scandals during those card games. We were probably considered lower middle class on an economic scale, but we never did without and had the greatest childhood ever.

It was 2007 when we started noticing Mom's decline. She was sixty-seven years old. It wasn't a slow decline. This disease took her body at a good steady pace. Her balance was off, then her speech became broken. Soon she could only repeat what was spoken to her. She couldn't get her thoughts out, but she sure tried. She lost bladder control. Her hands were starting to turn in on her. It was two years later that we got the diagnosis of Lewy body dementia. We had already suspected it from our research.

Dad desperately wanted to keep her at home, but it became way too much for him or any of us to handle. We moved her to a nursing care facility. By this time, Mom was confined to a wheelchair which she could move with her feet. Her speech was gone except for some choice outbursts. We had never heard this lady say a curse word ever, but she could sure spit some out now with great emotion behind them. She lost the use of her hands and, soon after that, the ability to move the wheelchair on her own. It wasn't long before she became bedridden.

It was the physical part of this disease that took Mom. Her body shut down piece by piece. The hardest part was the loss of speech. I already mentioned how much Mom loved to talk. She always knew what was going on around her, but she couldn't join in. She always knew us. She might have ignored us, but she knew us. When a grandchild would walk into her room, she would light up. She never lost her smile or her sense of humor. She was even laughing with us a few days before she died. Four years after we noticed the first symptoms, she went to Heaven.

Mom (Grandmom) had seven grandchildren whom she adored: Morgan, Ty, J.W., Jody, Jared, Christy, and Jason. She missed their graduations, their weddings, and now their children. She now has ten great-grandchildren: Beckham, Hudson, John Walker, Teagan, Emma Grace, Emma Jay, Payton, Lane, Gabby, and Emerson, plus one on the way. Oh, how she would have loved them!

We will never understand how this good, loving mom was taken from us so soon, but we know she is in Heaven. We are sure she is talking while hanging out with family and friends at a campsite playing cards. Knowing Mom, she probably has Conway Twitty on one side and Charlie Pride on the other making them both sing.

Until we see you again, Mom,

Your family

About the Authors: LeAnn Morgan Miller is in her 34th year as an English teacher. She has been married to her husband, Gary, for thirty-three years. They have two children and two grandchildren. They live in New Boston, Texas.

Jan Morgan Alexander and her husband, Jason, live in Bearden, Arkansas. They have four children and three grandchildren plus one on the way. Jan was always the most hands-on with Mom's care. She is now spending a lot of time caring for our dad.

Mother, Sister, the Best Pieces of Me
Melissa Klaeb

Pamela Joyce Klaeb was officially diagnosed with young-onset Alzheimer's disease in 2013 in her mid-fifties. She passed away in December 2020, surrounded by those she held most dear.

"She's my sister!" my mom boldly proclaimed to the pharmacist, as I was paying for some medications at the counter. Slightly startled, the pharmacist and I looked up at each other and exchanged a quick, knowing glance – the kind I'd begun to exchange more frequently with grocery clerks and passersby these days, when my mom made out-of-place remarks, apropos of nothing.

Just weeks before, she had commented to her dentist that I was indeed, her daughter. At the time, I couldn't understand her newfound obsession with declaring our relationship to anyone we came into contact with. We were several years into her journey with early-onset Alzheimer's disease, and the correct classifications of me as "daughter" left me hopeful, while the others nicked my insides. Was she feeling her memory slip away and simply trying to place me? Were the statements meant for others? Or did they serve to convince herself?

Four years prior, before her diagnosis, she was still working as an RN at our local hospital, and I had begun to volunteer on a rehab floor, to get experience before entering Physical Therapy school. Some days we had lunch together in the cafeteria. One afternoon as she slowly sipped on a bowl of cheddar broccoli soup and I picked away at my smattering of dry veggies and beans from the salad bar, a nurse she worked with approached us.

"Hi Pam, working the Saturday shift again I see," he commiserated.

"Yeah, but I'm here with my daughter!" she beamed.

"Daughter? I thought you two were sisters!"

Her face brightened with a glow I'd seen wash over her in moments of pride. When I scored a goal in water polo and looked over into the stands. When my brother was hooded on his law school graduation stage at NYU. When I told her I was considering a career in healthcare. And now, when we had been deemed *sisters*.

Like most mothers and daughters, our relationship had been a tenuous one, especially in my teenage years. We bickered often, but in my infinite wisdom more than a decade later, I realize now what often kindled our contentions was my need for autonomy and her desire to be best friends. She often received the hurtful blows of a stubborn, willful teenage girl who knew not the pain she inflicted. When I went away to college, a switch flipped. Overcome with a sickness for home, I needed her more than I had ever before. She held space for my sobs over the phone, when I could find a private spot to finally let my emotions escape. She mailed me cards for every occasion, and no occasion at all. When I moved out of the dorms and into my first apartment, she gifted me with a scrapbook of handwritten recipes she made when I was growing up. Her famous cashew chicken and Christmas holly cookies.

I shared details of my life with her I hadn't before. About the boy I started to date and fell in love with. How scared I was at the uncertainty of my future and frustration that I couldn't decide on a clear path. My need to be separate from her was replaced by a longing for closeness. She treated this transformation with gentleness, never prying for details, but accepting every offering with patience and joy.

As sometimes accompanies age, a wisdom began to form in me in those years. I began to appreciate my mom in a way kids and teenagers almost never can. I saw her kindness – not only in the cards she wrote – but in the way she rarely turned a charity down for money, and no matter how pressed for time, always returned the shopping cart. I reveled in her skills as a nurse, and how calm she remained in emergencies. I delighted in her literary prowess, her ability to finish the Sunday crosswords, and her confidence to do them in pen.

"Sisters," she smiled at me, as her coworker walked away from our table. I gave a quick smile back and finished up my lunch. In the moment, I hadn't paused to consider why that comment had brought her such joy. I'm sure part of it was the acknowledgment that she looked young enough to be the sister of a twenty-three-year-old. But I know it was more than that. Sisters brought forth a new possibility of closeness. Of telling secrets and forming alliances. It bridged a gap that had spaced us for so long.

Through the years of her Alzheimer's disease, I have been many people to her. Daughter, sister, friend. A hard-to-place familiar face. I'm glad at times I could be a sister for her. But I'm more grateful to be her daughter, because of what I now know so clearly – that the best pieces of me are the ones I can trace back to her. And the identity she was proudest of was, Mom.

Five short months after her passing, I became a mom as well. My grief widened, as I now longed for her guidance and gentle reassurance, stumbling through the early mornings and sleepless nights of caring for a newborn. Unbeknownst to us both, she had prepared me well for this new role, by allowing me to care for her in her final years. And her legacy of motherhood will live on through me. My boy and I will make brownies and lick the spoon with the batter. We will get burgers on Friday nights and watch the bunnies in the park. We will curl up and read books at night together. He will get cards in the mail from me when he goes off to college. He will be so loved, because I was loved so well.

About the Author: Melissa is the Director of Education for Alzheimer's Orange County in Irvine, California, an organization she became involved with after receiving invaluable support during her mother's journey with Alzheimer's. She cared for her mother for 10 years during her time with dementia. Melissa is now learning the ropes of motherhood herself with a new baby boy. She can also be found reading and writing, enjoying great meals with good company, and spending time near beautiful bodies of water. Please follow Melissa on Twitter @MelissaKlaeb and on Instagram @alzthingsconsidered.

The Eighth Street Dairy
Karen Malena

Karen's mother Eileen began to exhibit symptoms of dementia around 2010. Karen's father, Richard, who adored his wife, took care of her until his passing in September of 2016. Karen's mom passed away only ten months later in July of 2017 from Alzheimer's related complications.

I see Mom standing behind the counter of the small hometown Mom-and-Pop store—the Eighth Street Dairy that she and Dad owned for a time. It was there she was happiest. There, that she blossomed.

Born into a family in the late nineteen-thirties, she'd been told she was unwanted and unloved—a mistake. But the woman in the Eighth Street Dairy is no mistake. She is here for a reason.

The glass on the door of the milk coolers gleams and shines; the countertops of the sit-down lunch bar are wiped clean and ready for whoever the day brings into the store. All of the potato chip racks are stacked with every crispy flavor; the bread aisle stuffed with bright packaging, soft loaves, and buns; the soda pop chills.

Mom greets the regulars and she knows not only their names but their stories because she always says that everyone has a story to tell. The lady over there has an abusive husband; the one over there is going through health issues. That mean schoolteacher is lonely and only acts tough as if trying to impress everyone. But Mom sees through the façade and she gives and she loves and she reaches and she touches more lives than she may ever know.

When Mom lost her sister in 1968, she had a breakdown of sorts and there were times she didn't know who she was. But she always knew me and she called me her shining star. She said I was always the one thing she could come back to. When she tried suicide—when everything seemed so bleak—God saved her not only for me but for a future baby--my brother--a baby she was told to abort but would not.

At the Dairy, Mom sips her steaming cup of coffee and chats with a best friend from childhood. They laugh about the handsome customer, who just left the store, and they giggle like schoolgirls and they are young again without a care in the world.

Then another young man walks in—the one who Mom favors and loves. She treats him like family; she understands his home life and problems. She embraces him with her words and deeds and this man will never forget her.

She carefully counts out bags of penny candy: Swedish fish, flying saucers, gumballs, candy lipstick, licorice, and more. The hordes of children will soon come when their school day is over and she is ready with sacks of one hundred of each item. She thinks of them as hers these kids; a little brood of young chicks and she is the hen of this little fold and she lovingly cares for them, smiles at them, and gives of her time.

Her face lights up when the love of her life walks through the door after his day of work. Dad greets her with a kiss and Mom tells him about her day; about the new people she's met and how everyone's story is so unique.

#

Does she realize just how unique her story is though? How could a woman who not only had a mental breakdown but then a cardiac arrest ever sum up what her life has been about? Her heart issue came after Mom gained a huge amount of weight during the time before she was well and whole again; before her mind came back. The doctor had put her on water pills but he'd forgotten a slight detail: potassium. When Mom blanked out—when I heard her fall upstairs when I was a child and went running for Dad to tell him yet again something bad happened, how were we to know that this story would change more lives than ever?

When Mom awoke from resuscitation, she told Dad she wasn't afraid to die. She saw something beautiful and felt something wonderful. There's so much more she said, and a feeling of complete love, unlike anything this world has to offer. She felt as if she mattered and she did. She took this with her and told this story up to the end of her good life, even to a pastor in the nursing home only a month before we lost her.

#

Other young people come in to the dairy and they tell Mom secrets—things they would never tell another soul. She understands them though some are so rough around the edges and hardened and beat down. She knows what that is like from a childhood of fear from a drunken, abusive father. She cries for the child inside each of them as she heals from her own battle scars. She teaches forgiveness to them as she's had to forgive her mother for not loving her enough and her father for his many sins. She lets go and shows them how to let go and they love her for it and many remember her forever.

#

She lost two babies in a short time when I was young. She was told that another pregnancy could be devastating. But Mom, my brave mother told the doctor that she would have this later-in-life baby or die trying. And my brother was born and loved and was raised with a good heart by two parents and a sister who adored him.

#

Mom worries over her little boy when she works at the store. She keeps an eye on him as he makes new friends and she protects him best she can from what is bad in the world. She takes his friends into her little fold and they spend hours, oh so many hours at our house and they eat our dinner and feel more like family than friends. We all love them and they love us and our circle grows yet wider and larger.

When the time comes for the dairy to be sold, I know a piece of Mom goes with it. Yet as years progress, people come to her and say how she helped mold them and change their lives. If it wasn't for you, they say. . . She cries but they are happy tears but she is humble and does not let this change her simple, good heart. She's a soul with a body, my mother. A beautiful butterfly who has emerged from a cocoon of sadness into the light of a bright new day.

Another business venture will follow: an antique shop. They sometimes write it as 'Shoppe' so that it is fancy, but nothing is fancy about Mom. She fits in where the neighborhood is a bit snobbish and once again doesn't change who she is or make pretenses. She is one-of-a-kind and real. They like her for this in this village of the wealthy. They accept her. She gives more than she receives sometimes but she doesn't complain. Being a businesswoman compliments my mother. She has a mind like a steel trap as they say.

Later in life that mind begins to falter. The businesses are gone and with them some of the memories. But that one young man she loved oh so much from her time at the Eighth Street Dairy remembers her. I have re-met him and again he tells me how much my mother meant to him. As I whisper his name to Mom two days before we lose her, she smiles, sighs, and repeats his name to me. She will take a small piece of all of those lives she touched with her where we cannot follow.

About the Author: With a vivid imagination, the lessons learned in childhood, and the love of a close, Italian family, Karen began writing heartfelt, inspirational fiction novels, one which closely follows many of the conversations she and her mother shared through the years: *Reflections From my Mother's Kitchen: A Journey of Healing and Hope.*

When her mother began showing signs of Alzheimer's-type dementia in the last several years, Karen once again stepped into the role of caregiver for her aging parents along with the help of a wonderful brother. It was watching the love between her parents into the golden years which inspired her fiction novels about dementia: *Love Woven in Time*, and *Love Finds a Way.*

Karen has been active mentoring young writers, speaking at local libraries, schools, and care facilities. Recently she became a member of AlzAuthors, a loving community of writers dedicated to encouraging caregivers and family members of loved ones with dementia and Alzheimer's. Karen is a passionate advocate for the elderly. Her walk with God has given her the inspiration to blog about losing her parents and their family's journey from grief to healing and other heartfelt, encouraging tales.

Several of Karen's stories were recently chosen by Guidepost's sister magazines for publication. "The Earrings" appeared in *Mysterious Ways* magazine, "The Memory Blanket," in *Angels on Earth,* and "Merry Christmas Mom and Dad," as well as a few others.

She has written several other books, *Piggy*, a fun cat story which showcases friendship and carries an anti-bullying message, and *Sound of Silence*, a cautionary dystopian tale about a society forbidden to utter the spoken word. Karen also is part of an anthology about rescue cats, entitled *Rescued Two: The Healing Stories of Twelve Cats Through Their Eyes*.

Karen is a member of Pittsburgh East Scribes writer's group and Ligonier Valley Writers. She lives in Pennsylvania with her husband.

You can find her heartfelt blogs at *The Finch's Nest: Inspirational Stories,* http://karenmalena.blogspot.com and her books on Amazon. You can also find her on Facebook, Twitter, Instagram, Good Reads and Booksie.

Two Wheels and a Chocolate Bar
Elissa Boreham

Dave was assessed with cognitive impairment in 2016 at age 79, and later formally diagnosed with Alzheimer's in March 2017. His condition declined quickly, further complicated by diabetes. He resided in a long-term care facility until his passing in July 2019.

His name was Boreham. Dave Boreham, and he was my dad.

My father was a huge James Bond fan, so I felt this opening was very appropriate. We didn't have a lot of things in common but a mutual love of all things 007 was most certainly one of them. When a new James Bond movie was released, he and I would almost always see it together. In fact, the last one we saw together was *Spectre* and my son came along with us too, which was great.

My dad was a very private person and not very forthcoming about a great many things. I think some of that came from his very proper English background and his conservative demeanor which didn't really allow him to share much with his kids. He would give us little bits of information like breadcrumbs, so you'd have to try and follow the trail.

Occasionally you would get an answer, sometimes the one you wanted, sometimes not. Most of the time you would follow up and he would immediately change the subject and then never tell you. I remember this drove me crazy when I was younger, but as I grew into adulthood, I realized it was just part of who he was.

My dad had a very fractured childhood. His father abandoned his family, leaving his mother and three children to fend for themselves following the end of the Second World War. It was very difficult but eventually she managed to start over and met my grandfather Reg. They later married and went on to have two more children. There was a very large age difference between the three original children and the two half-siblings. My dad's stepfather and his mother moved to Canada while my father remained in the UK.

He spent a short time in the Royal Air Force serving his country and developing his love of aircraft. It was during this time that he met my mother. They married when she was just 19 and he was 23 on March 18, 1961, and soon after relocated to Canada.

My sister was born February 21, 1962, and just like that my dad became a parent. I don't think either of them was really prepared for having kids so quickly, but things happen and six years later I arrived on January 1, 1968.

My dad worked in a bank for most of his career, and he loved to work on DIY projects. It was a real change of pace to work with his hands and explore his creative side.

He was also amazing at photography, and it brought him great joy throughout his life. Somehow, he could look at an object and capture it at different angles that weren't obvious at first glance to someone else, but it would result in some unique images that I loved. Many of these now decorate my home since his passing in 2019.

One of his other passions was cycling. He'd done some competitive racing in his youth but his love of riding continued well into his early 70s. He was always happy zipping around on his bike, heading over to the Toronto Islands on the ferry, and spending the day exploring or catching some sun on the beach.

The need to keep busy following his retirement, and earn a little extra money was super important for his wellbeing. As a result, he worked part-time at a few different car dealerships in the city, driving cars from place to place for customers. He loved it. The opportunity to try out different vehicles and not buy them was a perfect role for him.

Eventually, as he got older, he was asked to drive the courtesy shuttle instead, but he still thoroughly enjoyed it and the social aspect was really great for him.

Though my father had a good circle of friends for many years, he found it challenging as inevitably some of the older ones passed away and he found fewer and fewer people interested in getting out and about.

Thankfully he had a female companion for many, many years and I was very grateful she was in his life, especially when he started to have cognitive challenges. When he was still living alone, she made meals for him so he wouldn't have to cook. She was his rock and never wavered in her love, even as his disease progressed and he moved to a different town. She always came to see him, armed with his favourite sweet treats – a Boston cream doughnut or chocolate bar, and his double-double Tim Hortons coffee. Music was something that energized him and was ever-present in his life. Rarely would you see my father and there would not be some form of music on in the background. Though he loved many different genres, it is probably jazz and some Brazilian music that most reminds me of my dad. He loved João Gilberto, Astrud Gilberto, and Stan Getz performing "The Girl from Ipanema." I remember watching the movie *Eat, Pray, Love* recently and hearing that song in the film made me smile.

I miss my dad very much, but it's comforting to know that whenever I hear a certain song, see a plane fly overhead, rewatch a Monty Python movie I've seen umpteen times. or indulge in a Mars bar (his favourite), it's like he's right here with me. I love you, Dad.

About the Author: Elissa Boreham is a single, self-employed mother of two, and lives about an hour away from Toronto, Canada. Her youngest child is autistic, and both her father (passed July 2019) and mother have had Alzheimer's and dementia. Inspired by the caregiving journey she has been on and wanting to pass along some knowledge, her website, blog, and podcast www.68spidrs.ca were created. A work in progress, she enjoys being able to share her thoughts with others on a similar journey. You can reach Elissa through her website and on Twitter, @ElissaBoreham.

The Traveller Extraordinaire
Elissa Boreham

Diana was assessed with cognitive impairment in 2018 at age 77, which was then diagnosed as vascular dementia and aphasia in May 2019. Her condition has rapidly declined, and she is currently living in an assisted living facility.

My mother loved to visit new places, so it was a natural fit that she ended up working in the travel industry for most of her working life.

She was born in the early part of the Second World War in a small town near Nottingham, in the United Kingdom. The eldest of two children, her father was a very emotionally distant man, so as a result, she was extremely close to her mother who showered her with love and affection.

She met my father at a dance at the Palais, and they were immediately smitten with one another. On March 18th, 1961 they married when she was only 19 years old. It's hard to imagine nowadays getting married so young, especially as my son is 19 and he's definitely not ready for marriage, but at that time it was not that unusual.

Following the wedding, they moved to Canada, where my father's parents had already relocated sometime prior. My mother was newly married, in a strange country and shortly thereafter found herself pregnant with my older sister Sarah, who was born February 21st, 1962.

A lot of changes for a very young woman, but she took it in stride.

Never one to sit still, it always seemed like we moved about every 4 years, usually because my mother was ready for a change or dissatisfied with the house or location. Eventually, this wandering spirit ended up taking our family back to the UK in 1974.

My parents both loved the idea of owning their own business, so they purchased a beautiful old period home with a small post office and general store attached. Located in the small Welsh village of Guilsfield, it was a wonderful place to raise a family, albeit a little dull for my older sister and me, but we managed to make our own entertainment.

The business flourished, and we took lots of family trips around the UK, and to places like Spain and Tunisia. Everything seemed perfect, and it was one of the happiest times of my life.

Unfortunately, things were not as untroubled as I had believed them to be, and eventually, my parents sold the business and separated. My dad moved back to Canada and my mother, sister, and I stayed in the UK and moved to Long Eaton, a small town where my mother grew up and my grandmother still resided.

My mother managed to get a job as a travel agent in a nearby town. It did not pay very well, and with a mortgage, car, and kids she was really struggling. About two years later during a visit with my dad, they decided to try again. Unfortunately, the early 1980s were a tough time economically in the UK and he was unable to find a job, and just like that we moved again and were back in Canada.

We were once again in Toronto and my parents bought a major fixer-upper and set to work renovating. The physical work and planning of what project to tackle next were good distractions, but it was clear my mother was not truly contented. I am not sure if my dad didn't notice or just chose to ignore her mood swings.

She continued working in the tourism industry and travelled the globe. The frequent trips abroad were a welcome respite from the unhappiness in her marriage and she always returned in a much better mood than when she left.

Eventually, my parents separated again and finally divorced. My mother blossomed in her newfound freedom and began a journey of discovering who she was and what made her happy.

It was wonderful to be around my mother as her joie de vivre was infectious. She loved having dinner parties and entertaining her friends. She enjoyed trying new things and pushing the boundaries of her previously conservative background. There was always a lot of laughter. It was during this time that we were not only mother and daughter, but we also became friends.

My mother's work allowed us to visit some incredible places together. Egypt, Greece, and Malta were vacations I will always remember and I am so grateful I had the chance to visit them with her.

An avid gardener and pet lover, we always had dogs and cats growing up and, every home we lived in had an amazing garden. She found such joy getting her fingers into the soil and turning a patch of sparse grass into such a beautiful place to spend time. When my mother stopped working on her garden was when I really knew that something had changed.

When I think of my mum this is how I see her, even now. A beautiful woman, with sparkling eyes and an easy laugh, wearing her sun hat and shades and digging up weeds in her happy place.

Dementia may have stripped her of so many things, but it cannot take away all the love we have for her, now and always.

About the Author: Elissa Boreham is a single, self-employed mother of two, and lives about an hour away from Toronto, Canada. Her youngest child is autistic, and both her father (passed July 2019) and mother have had Alzheimer's and dementia. Inspired by the caregiving journey she has been on, and wanting to pass along some knowledge, her website, blog, and podcast www.68spidrs.ca were created. A work in progress, she enjoys being able to share her thoughts with others on a similar journey. You can connect with Elissa on her website and on Twitter, @ElissaBoreham.

Marathon Woman
Tony Copeland-Parker

Catherine was diagnosed with early-onset Alzheimer's in 2014 at the age of 53. She is now in the moderate range in terms of the progression of the disease however she is still enjoying life to the fullest.

Marathons don't define her but do describe her. The same determination and grit which is required to complete 26.2 miles, on foot, nonstop, in a race, have been her guiding light through the trials and tribulations of her current condition. April 2014, she was handed the detailed 29-page report from her neurologist that described her condition as early-onset Alzheimer's or like condition. They say you really don't know for sure until the autopsy so the three letters, EOA, will work for us, for now. We could have done some more expensive testing to rule out other word-salad ailments, but how we tackle the daily challenges would still be the same.

Catherine Elizabeth Popp grew up amongst her four highly competitive siblings when even having a meal was a competitive sport. At the dinner table, you got what you could and sharing was a personal foul. That attitude made its way to the football field for the three boys, with swimming and track, for all five of them. Catherine's deceased dad, Tom, who succumbed to vascular dementia in his 70's, threw her in the pool at six and simply said, "swim or drown." She has been doing all the strokes possible ever since then in this race we call life, her favorite being the butterfly because of its level of difficulty.

As a child, Catherine swam like a fish, earning a multitude of ribbons and trophies that had to share space with her sister's awards in the bedroom they shared. As an adult one sport was not enough for her so biking and running were added for one simple reason; because she could. For Catherine, winning was not as important as doing. The feeling of pushing herself was what made her feel the most comfortable.

Catherine is determined to live a full life even though there are many parts of it she may not clearly remember without a reminder. She definitely does not need to be reminded of the motorcycle ride she made to and from the west coast from her hometown in Indiana. She soundly repeats that story every time she sees or even hears a motorcycle go by, her smile as wide as ever, which includes her beautiful, sparkling, blue eyes. Catherine made the trip with a friend, each of them riding their own bike. It was an experience Catherine will never forget.

A college degree was something Catherine always wanted to earn and for her, no time was like the present. At the age of 32, she put the plan together to get it done in five years. That meant working at night, tossing packages, some the size of her, at UPS, and going to school during the day. Many thought that was a daunting task, but for her, it was just a way of life. That's the way Catherine approached everything, with enthusiasm and a detailed plan.

Catherine's daughter was in high school at this time so throw in taking care of her daughter, meal preparations, and sleeping, along with working full-time and going to college. My head swims with thoughts of how she was able to do this all by herself! It does explain how she can handle the daily changes to her mind and how it currently processes information. This gives a picture of how determined Catherine has always been, even now. Just like the attitude she takes towards running a marathon, she just puts her head down, puts one foot in front of the other, and never gives up.

Catherine and her daughter are only 18 years apart in age and she did the majority of the parenting all by herself. I still remember, to this day, when we first met, Catherine told me that she did not need a man and she went through most of her life proving it in her own way. She lost her husband when she was in her 30's after only being married for a year. That is when marathoning came into her life like a guiding light. Her oldest brother took her under his wing to save her from the spiral of despair and they began the journey of running a marathon in all 50 states. They began with 5K, 10K, and 13.1 mile half marathon races as they worked up to the 26.2 mile marathon distance at the Chicago Marathon in 1997.

I met Catherine, by chance, as I overheard her talking to others about running marathons. I joined in on the conversation and I knew in an instant that she was the one. Her stories took me back to my years growing up in New York watching the New York City Marathon on TV. I dreamed of one day running in that race, not as one of the elite runners, the multitude of cameras following their every step, but one of the masses of humanity that followed way behind. When Catherine talked about running a marathon, determination oozed from her pores and I knew then that no matter what, she would always land on her feet.

I convinced Catherine to train me to run the New York City Marathon in 2000 and as they say, the rest is history. My thoughts were like most that complete a marathon, one and done, but she had other plans. Not sure if they included me but I was willing to tag along, as long as I could. Race after race became more daunting to me but seemed effortless to her.

In 2001 after 9/11, the Transportation Security Administration was spooled up in response, and Catherine, with an extensive scheduling background, joined forces as a Scheduling Operations Supervisor. She was responsible for the scheduling of all the agents in three airports in Kentucky. She was in her element, with everyone loving her even if they did not get exactly what they had hoped for on their daily schedule. She had a way to make everyone feel like they were her best friend and that she sincerely had all their best interests at heart.

Dogs, anything furry, and babies are her true weakness. Catherine took care of our two 90 pound dogs with ease, often having to referee between the two. Her days often started at 5:00 AM with these two highly rambunctious dogs. They frequently trained with her, with the Doberman completing a marathon with Catherine. My dog which was a Weimaraner had little interest in running that distance. He was more of a sprinter from one fire hydrant to the next.

I did take Catherine off course when it came to completing her goal of getting a marathon done in each state plus DC, when we went to Athens, Greece, to run our first international marathon as my 50th birthday present to her. We went in 2010 which was a big deal for the Athens Marathon. It was merely 2500 years prior, in 490 BC, when

Pheidippides ran from Marathon to Athens and later died. We were no longer getting faster, ourselves, so when the thought of us finishing the race in over 5 hours became apparent we grabbed each other's hand and sprinted across the finish line. Me being over a foot taller than Catherine, the finisher photo had her completely airborne as if I was pulling a rag doll. The timing clock overhead read 4 hours and 59 minutes.

During conversations with others about our running prowess, Catherine was always quick to point out three things that separated the two of us.

One, that her fastest marathon time is eight minutes faster than mine. Catherine's is 3 hours and 49 minutes.

Two, that she actually qualified for the Boston Marathon. A runner has to accomplish a previous marathon within a specified time limit for their age and gender. I, however, donated to charity to get the opportunity to run the coveted marathon.

Three, that she has run 15 more marathons than me.

These three points will forever be.

One of Catherine's greatest accomplishments is her only daughter. She has grown into a successful lawyer who runs a law firm with her husband. Together they have raised three fantastically ambitious children who all love to run which gives Catherine much joy. Before her diagnosis, they lived close by and she would visit them often to participate in many of their daily activities.

We enjoyed the adventures of travel to foreign lands as we would go on race-cations to places we could only imagine years prior. These international races slowed down the pace of Catherine's goal of finishing a marathon in all 50 states, but it was something she kept a keen eye on. Goal setting is an integral part of who she is.

I started to notice that she was not on her usual A-game, and she would begin asking me to repeat plans jointly made. Catherine got a new boss and he was a "shake things up" type of guy. Routine was now her cornerstone so he made life at work more difficult, which, in turn, made it easier to help Catherine realize that something was just not right. To help protect her government job I made sure she saw and documented visits to the neurologist so that a simple firing by her new boss would not sweep the now obvious problem under the rug.

She was able to get a nice severance package including a timely pension with health care. Social security followed suit with a disability determination. The diagnosis, as it often does, changed our lives, as it does all, but our reaction to the news was counter-intuitive.

We both retired, sold our home, and became nomads running all over the world. Catherine's resilience or reserve, as it were, is anything athletic, so we combined that with our love of travel. Together we have visited 81 different countries and run at least a half marathon in 35 of them with these events covering all seven continents. Catherine has completed 83 marathons, one Iron Man Competition, a 50 miler Ultra Marathon and many races and triathlons of various distances. Prior to her diagnosis, she completed four of the six major marathons, New York,

Chicago, Boston, and London. Since her diagnosis, she was able to achieve the other two in Tokyo and Berlin.

In October 2020 I had the pleasure to once again cross the finish line hand-in-hand with Catherine but this time it was when she completed her 50th state, in Narragansett, Rhode Island. She now has a fourth accomplishment to hold over my head and to brag to others about, but now, I doubt she will ever do so.

We celebrated Catherine's 60th birthday, along with her 86 year old, highly energetic mother, at the Kentucky Derby which falls on Catherine's birthday every five to six years. She was quick to remind us that she was also there when she turned 21 but did not actually see a single race. I wonder why.

Catherine's new goal is to finish a half marathon in all 50 states plus DC and as of September 2021, she has 40 of them under her feet with five more, for a total of 45, planned by the end of the year. Catherine expects to reach her goal in spring, 2022. You can follow her continued adventures at RunningwithCat.com and read all about our life as nomads in my book, *Running All Over The World, Our Race Against Early Onset Alzheimer's*.

About the Author: Tony Copeland-Parker was a professional pilot/manager for thirty-seven years, the last twenty-seven with United Parcel Service. His last job had him managing pilots and flying B757/767-type aircraft all over the world. You can find Tony on Facebook, Twitter and Instagram or through his website http://runningwithcat.com.

The Good Soldier
Miriam Galindo

Henry Brady Brown was born on December 19, 1938. He died of complications due to Alzheimer's disease on February 25, 2016. He was a devoted husband to his wife of more than 50 years, Erika Salditt Brown, who died a few years later on October 3, 2020. He is survived by his five children.

My Dad would be mortified if he found out I am writing this essay about him. He was a quiet, unassuming, sensitive soul who despised self-aggrandizement. Everyone who knew him can attest to that. What most people did not know, however, is how Dad enlisted in the Army. This is the story I want to share with you today.

Let me start by describing our Dad. To say he was a man of few words is inaccurate. A natural, literary genius, he believed that the most important things in life transcended the constraints of spoken language. These things included intangible or sacred concepts like God, love, truth, justice, responsibility, courage, hope, and faith. Truly, Dad was a master at conveying these concepts without using any words at all.

When we five kids were little, the highlight of our day was bedtime. We didn't have a television, iPhone, iPad, or video games to entertain us. We didn't need them. We had our Dad! After dinner, we would hurry through our baths, brush our teeth, and gather around the kitchen table in our pajamas to watch Dad draw a picture. Thereafter, we would settle into our beds and listen to old-time radio shows until we drifted off to sleep. Like the dramatic scripts of old-time radio shows, we never knew what to expect from our Dad's drawings, nor would Dad ruin the suspense by telling us. We just watched in hushed silence as the plot emerged. Looking back, I can see that his drawings conveyed a theme which was not consciously understood to us at the time. In his drawings, hope endured: nothing was impossible, every problem had a solution, there was no fear, good always conquered evil, and we innocent children always emerged the heroes.

When I was about four years old, for example, there lived a great big dog in our neighborhood. His name was Charlie and he terrorized us with his great big bark. Dad validated our fears by drawing a picture of Charlie. But in Dad's drawing, Charlie was neither big nor scary and the spell of Charlie's tyrannical reign soon lost its grip over us forevermore. Another time, my brother Daniel developed a fear after overhearing a radio news story about a rash of robberies in New Orleans. Dad acknowledged Daniel's fears by drawing a picture of the robber in the act of stealing Dad's transistor radio. But in Dad's version, three-year-old Daniel is bravely pointing a steady finger at the burglar and saying with poised authority, "Stop Wobber!"

When Daniel was afraid of sleeping alone because a monster lived under his bed, Dad drew a picture of Daniel looking under his bed, and yes indeed, there was a monster living under his bed. But it turned out the monster wasn't trying to scare Daniel; the monster was simply hungry and wanted a sandwich. What's more, my brother Tormay and I are laughing and pointing at him because the monster is not wearing any pants.

My Dad's illustrations allowed us kids to transcend every fear, obstacle, and barrier. Through his art, my brother Tormay secured a high-dollar Invicta Chronograph diving watch, built a sports car in the garage, and took a ferry ride by himself to Algiers. My brother Daniel expertly flew several WWII bomber airplanes, mastered underwater scuba diving, defended himself in a lion's den with a loaded bazooka, and drove a camouflaged war tank. My brothers and I ice-skated on a frozen pond despite never seeing snow in real life. And when Superman became incapacitated by a piece of kryptonite, it was my little brother Aaron, or maybe Sebastian Joseph, who picked up the deadly rock and successfully disposed of it in a trashcan.

Dad's own line-up of superheroes included missionaries and saints who got themselves into some gnarly situations. One of Dad's favorites was Sir Isaac Jogues a Jesuit priest who left the comforts of his bourgeois family to serve the Iroquois and Huron people located in what we now know as Auriesville, New York. Jogues was a hard-core honey badger. He did not shy away from adversity at all; rather, he stared it down while enduring unspeakable torture and brutality. Many of us would view this life as something from which we would surely escape. But when Jogues was given an opportunity to go home, he chose to return to that mess of a mission field where he was ultimately martyred by one of the most ruthless and notorious New World gangs of the 17th century, the Mohawks. Dad so admired Jogues that he had all of us kids read the biography *Saint in the Wilderness* which, if you have not read it, will completely freak you out. The story not only redefines courage but will also make you think, "What in the heck empowers a person to say 'yes' to something like that?"

As we grew older and moved to California, Dad's drawings became more sophisticated both in content and drawing style. One collection conceived by Dad in the Spring of 1978 is especially noteworthy – a comic strip entitled *The Adventures of Jim Geronimo*. Dr. Jim Geronimo was a scientist at Cal Tech. Not surprisingly, he looked a lot like our Dad except he had a full head of perpetually tousled hair. In the opening scene, we see Dr. Geronimo bravely descending into a sewer pipe to battle an alien from outer space. While in the sewer pipe, Jim Geronimo is struck from behind and left for dead in the watery sewage, face down, as the alien monster absconds with Jim's beloved Mary Deer via an awaiting spaceship. The comic strip series follows Dr. Geronimo's determination to leave earth and find Mary Deer wherever she may be. In his determination, Geronimo single-handedly develops a blueprint for a rocket ship which will propel him from earth to outer space. But building it is one thing; paying for it is quite another. From his rotary dial phone, Dr. Geronimo solicits various people for funding including the President of the United States. Everyone, including the President, says no. Finally, Dr. Geronimo flies to Houston, Texas, to visit an elderly friend, Miss Ladijane Livewright. Without question, the sole heiress to a multi-billion dollar estate of Augustus Livewright's Atomic Fuel fortune gives Dr. Geronimo **everything** she owns and downsizes her palatial home to a single room at the YWCA.

Two important scenes come next. In the first scene, Dr. Geronimo wakes up from a bad dream the night before the start of his mission. The mood is somber as if Dr. Geronimo is suddenly overcome by the gravity of what his mission entails. He gets out of bed, turns on his desk lamp, and writes his last will and testament, leaving all his earthly possessions to his bumbling engineer friend, Professor Max Gorki. In another scene, his elderly benefactor Miss Livewright is watching a televised newscast of Dr. Geronimo's journey into outer space. The mood is somber as if she is suddenly overcome by the gravity of what this mission truly means. She turns off the television and opens a thick book to read the following words on a page:

> *I will take the wings of morning and dwell in the utmost parts of the sea.*

Unbeknownst to us kids at the time, the passage is from Psalm 139:9. The rest of the scripture essentially says, "God is there." In other words, whether Jim Geronimo travels to the highest heights of outer space or plummets into the deepest part of the ocean, God will be there to guide him and strengthen him.

On the day Dr. Geronimo makes his ascent, he is in reciprocal communication with NASA. Initially, everything looks OK. But over time, NASA loses his signal and Geronimo loses theirs. He struggles to ration what little oxygen he has left down to 12%. Eventually, he simultaneously loses consciousness while also losing fuel.

The reader is left wondering if Jim Geronimo is dead or alive. For a long time thereafter, we kids wondered what happened next. Did Jim Geronimo die or is he still alive? Did he complete his mission or not? We begged our Dad to draw the end of the story, but Dad never did and being a man of few words--and in this case no words--he never told us what happened either.

Decades later, on April 29, 1998, Dad and I were working together on a project to replace my linoleum kitchen floor with tile. I had a gnawing feeling that today was the day I had to ask Dad all the questions I ever wanted to ask. My first question sought to clarify a terrifying account I had inadvertently overheard when I was six years old about Dad's former coworker who sustained a massive injury while working with Dad on an off-shore commercial saturation diving unit. My Dad's explanation was just as disturbing as I remembered, causing me to wonder what in the heck would drive a person to say "yes" to a job like that. Next, I asked my Dad a seemingly innocuous question: "Hey Dad. What do you want to do in the next 20 years?" I remember him standing at the kitchen window, his face reflecting the brilliant orange light of the setting sun as he silently considered his answer.

"I want to be a Soldier for Christ," he told me with a discernible catch of emotion in his throat. "I want to hear Him say, 'Well done, good and faithful servant. Enter into the Kingdom of God.'"

Dad then told me this story. It was 1975. He received a call that it was his time to go to work. For weeks prior, he dreaded receiving this call and when it finally came, he avoided responding to it until he had no choice but to leave home and dutifully board a dinghy headed toward an off-shore barge located in the deepest part of the sea. The dinghy drifted lethargically from the shoreline and, before long, brought him to the middle of nothing: He could see nothing in front of him, nothing to either side, and nothing behind him. For miles it seemed, there was nothing but the oppressive gloom of an endless, hopeless sea. To make matters worse, the water was so turbulent that Dad became violently ill to the point of losing almost ten percent of his body weight due to severe dehydration. "This is it," he realized with incredulity. "I'm going to die." But just as he felt himself sinking into the depths of despair, a helicopter suddenly appeared in the sky and began to dramatically descend over the dinghy. It was a medical flight sent just for him. In true form, Dad's depiction of this harrowing account was radio-worthy, replete with the exhilarating sound effects of whirring helicopter blades set against a musical score of Wagner's *Die Walküre*. He ended with Psalm 18:16 (NIV) quoted barely above a whisper:

> *He reached down from on high and took hold of me;*
> *He drew me out of deep waters.*

"That is Christ," he said.

The profundity of Dad's pledge to be a Soldier for Christ became more perspicuous in the years to follow. Only years later did I realize that what appeared to be just an ordinary day of laying tile was really Dad's Garden of Gethsemane. It was the day his application to the Army was accepted and he was officially recruited as a Soldier for Christ. But it would be another eighteen years before he was deployed to another world to see Christ face to face and hear Him say, "Well done, good and faithful servant."

First, Dad needed to complete one more critical mission on earth. This mission would require Dad to bravely enter a sewer pipe, just like Jim Geronimo, and successfully emerge from the other side, wherever that might be. The pipe would be daunting in length, about 11 to 16 years long depending on who you asked, and it was called Alzheimer's disease. Upon his initial descent, everything would appear to be okay. But later in the journey, communication between NASA and the spaceship would be lost. His brain would play tricks on him. He would feel disoriented and start questioning his sense of direction. He would have to navigate his way through uncertainty without the benefit of a working control panel. At times, he would feel as if he was flailing against raging waters and walking through fire. At other times, he would wonder if "this is it. I'm going to die." And throughout all of this, there would be but one command to follow: "Do not be afraid, Soldier" (Isaiah 43:2, paraphrased):

> *When you pass through raging waters, the General, God Himself, will be with you;*
> *And those waters? They won't overflow you*
> *When you walk through the fire, you won't be scorched*
> *The flame will not burn you…*

In other words, Charlie the Dog is only a bark; he cannot bite you. The monster under the bed cannot get you and besides, he isn't wearing any pants. You will not drown even though it feels like it at times. You will not be burned. Even kryptonite cannot harm you. No matter what, just keep marching, Soldier, and in the end, you WILL see Christ face to face.

If someone presented that scenario to me, would I have the courage to enter that pipe? Would you? Could I behold the significance of my mission amidst bleak circumstances to say "yes" to a job like that? My Dad certainly did. And he marched with an indomitable spirit all the way to the end.

My brother Tormay and I were with Dad when he died. It was 2:27 a.m. We wanted nothing more than for Dad to fall asleep – no more struggle, no more discomfort. But Dad persisted relentlessly as if he was running the best marathon of his life. Tormay finally suggested that we download an old-time radio show on his iPhone, the same nightly radio shows we listened to as children when it was time for bed. Tormay placed the iPhone on Dad's chest where it played a full episode of *The Lone Ranger* from 1938. The announcer commenced with this familiar introduction:

> *In the early days...a masked man...rode the plains searching for truth and justice...Nowhere in the pages of history can one find a greater champion of justice! Return with us now to those thrilling days of yesteryear! From out of the past come the thundering hoofbeats of the great horse Silver! The Lone Ranger rides again!*

As my brother and I chatted over the dialogue, Dad's breathing became calmer and his facial expression relaxed to the point where he looked very much like the younger Dad we knew as children. At the culmination of the show, when the Lone Ranger shouts "Hi-Yo Silver away!" followed by the rousing rendition of the fourth movement of Rossini's *William Tell Overture*, Dad quietly exhaled his final breath as if falling into a peaceful sleep.

Later, I emailed my brother Daniel to assure him that Dad was now a Soldier of Christ and if God's Army was anything like earth's Army, they probably had a football team which was a good thing because Dad was an avid sports fanatic. Daniel responded that he had just returned from attending a University of Texas basketball game that morning. Texas called a timeout toward the end of the game during which the band played a song. And what do you suppose they played? The theme from the Lo-o-o-o-o-one Ranger.

So now you know how our Dad enlisted in God's Army as a Soldier for Christ. Dad's decision to reveal his final destination to me prior to diagnosis turned out to be an indispensable gift. It served to illuminate my path as caregiver during the darkest moments of his disease and bolstered me with an unwavering conviction to boldly march alongside Dad on his providential path. Today, I know with full confidence that Dad is exactly where he wanted to be as a most worthy servant and faithful soldier for Jesus Christ. Well done, Dad. Nowhere in the pages of history can one find a greater champion of truth, mercy, and justice. Hi-Yo Silver away!

About the Author: Miriam Galindo Psy.D., LCSW, RPT, MSN, RN, RPT is a practicing psychologist, social worker, play therapist, nurse, and long-time family caregiver for both her belated Dad and Mom. She has been a volunteer caregiver educator at Alzheimer's Orange County since 2016.

A Creative Helper
Jennifer Fink

Diane Marie (Ridge) Graham was born in 1943 in Alameda County California. She is the oldest of four siblings. Diane's grandmother suffered from dementia and her mother had vascular dementia. Diane was formally diagnosed with Alzheimer's disease in 2011 but this only served to confirm what the family already knew.

Writing about who Mom was before her diagnosis was more challenging than I expected. Because Mom had Alzheimer's for at least twenty years, it's hard to remember the "before" times. As I thought about who Mom was before her Alzheimer's, I discovered something about myself: We are more alike than I realized.

Referring to my mom as a creative helper hopefully starts painting the picture of who she was. Looking back, she had quite an exciting array of interests. She was what you think of as a typical 1960s housewife, managing the family, household, and the photography business her husband ran as a side business.

When I was a young child, Mom took up cake decorating and created beautiful birthday cakes for our family. Some were elaborate, while others we personalized for each of us. What I find funny and interesting was she never made the cakes from scratch. Mom baked cookies from scratch but never anything else. Cookie mixes weren't available in the mid-70s as far as I remember but I'm not sure she would have used them. Store-bought cookies were never a regular item in our home, the only exceptions being Fig Newtons and Oreos.

Remembering the holidays, Mom created holiday dresses for herself and me and my sister. For years we had matching Mommy & Me dresses. I'd love to be able to ask her why she stopped making them. Thinking about those matching dresses reminds me of how my mom would Christmas shop.

My sister and I are nearly five years apart in age and are opposites in personality. Mom's solution to Christmas shopping, if you can call it that, was to shop for one of us on one day and shop on a different day for the other. Her shopping style drove my dad crazy with the illogic of it all. It also wasn't unusual for Mom to forget what she bought or where she had stashed gifts. Could this have been a sign of her future Alzheimer's, or was it just a case of disorganization?

Mom decided to try oil painting. She took lessons and painted all types of landscapes and still life paintings for many years. We hung one of her paintings in her room in the memory care residence. I don't think she recognized it as something she created, but my sister and I assumed it would be soothing.

Mom always had some creative projects in the works. The most special was all the items she created for my wedding. Being a typical middle-class family, the price of some things such as bridal veils was outrageous. Due to Mom's extensive sewing background, she was aware that the materials needed weren't expensive. That's how we ended up creating my wedding veil. Mom added faux pearls, one by one, to my veil, adding a personal touch and making it more beautiful than any veil I could have purchased. In addition, Mom made the bridesmaids' dresses, the flower girl dresses, the junior bridesmaids' dresses, and the guys' cummerbunds and bow ties. Oh, and she re-hemmed the dress she bought for herself at Macy's. The hemming happened within twenty-four hours of the wedding.

Mom always claimed to work better under pressure. Unfortunately for us, her procrastination caused the rest of the household a lot of angst. The above example of her hemming her dress the DAY of my wedding is an excellent one. Organization wasn't her strong suit and there always seemed to be a lot of last minute running around, suddenly remembered gifts, or holiday meal side dishes. There was always a lot of chaos from her during the holidays. One thing I think I may have inherited from her was not allowing for extra time to get someplace or finish a project. Time just seems to get away from me and I suspect that she was the same way.

Mom carried on these creative traditions with her oldest granddaughter. They created a sweatshirt with a wreath made from painted hands stamped onto the fabric when my daughter was about five-years-old. One of my daughter's fondest memories is baking with her grandma. Laura claims that she learned all her cooking and creativity from her grandmother and me, her mom. Creativity runs in our family but Mom definitely helped Laura to blossom as an artist and a baker.

These memories only touch on Mom's creative side, but she was a caregiver and helper too. She was a full-time wife and mother, but she also assisted our dad with his side business. Dad photographed weddings, and Mom was responsible for completing the finished product. They made a good team.

Mom always took care of her family, friends, and community. Over the years she participated in band and swim team fundraisers. Every day she seemed to do something to care for those around her. As my sister and I entered our teenage years, Mom joined a women's service organization called Soroptimist. She was an active member from 1985 until she moved into the memory care residence in 2017. She had good friends who picked her up for the meetings when she could no longer drive. I am confident they would have continued to include her had she not lived in the opposite direction of the meeting place.

Even when she lived in the memory care residence, Mom always offered her help to others. Her offers of help were sweet and funny because, at that time, she wasn't able to help herself.

Taking this walk down memory lane reminds me of one last thing; Mom was a big fan of talk radio and TV talk shows. I wish she had been able to understand how I adapted that love of hers to the current technology by creating my podcast. A podcast is a more modern version of talk radio.

During the pandemic, I transitioned full-time to podcasting and changed my hobby to something Mom would have loved. I create greeting cards for friends and loved ones. For Halloween 2020, I took treats and handmade cards to the residents where Mom lived. I know that's something she would have participated in with me before her diagnosis.

We don't always appreciate our similarities to our parents. Hearing my mom's voice come out of our mouth can be funny and unsettling. However, despite those moments of "I can't believe I just said that," I'm glad that my similarities to my mom are there. I like to think I've taken her traits and modernized them. I guess only time will tell on that!

About the Author: Jennifer Graham Fink has been an entrepreneur all her life. From 1991-2005 she worked in the family photography business. When her parents retired she went on her own. In 2018 she started a podcast called "Fading Memories" to help support other Alzheimer's caregivers. Jennifer is also a Rotarian and a volunteer with the Alzheimer's Association Northern CA/Northern Nevada. She is married to John and they have one adult daughter and many Golden Retrievers. You can follow her on Twitter and LinkedIn at Jennifer Fink or Facebook and Instagram @AlzheimersPodcast.

Give Good Gifts: Lessons I Learned from My Uncle Brian
Paulette Sharkey

Brian was diagnosed with Alzheimer's disease in 2016 and died in 2018 at the age of 79. He is dearly missed by his family.

My Uncle Brian and his quiet partner, Russ, were together for more than 50 years but never married. They didn't speak openly about their relationship and many in my small tight-knit extended family, including my parents, believed they were simply friends and roommates. Russ had no family, so we gathered him up into ours.

I learned many lessons from Uncle Brian by watching him navigate the world with his big heart and gentle ways.

Give good gifts

Brian was a loving, generous presence throughout my childhood. He bought gifts for every birthday and Christmas, and sometimes for no reason at all. He took my brother and sister and me on special solo outings. For me, the most memorable was a Van Cliburn concert in Detroit in the mid-1960s when I was about twelve years old.

Cliburn had won the first International Tchaikovsky Piano Competition in Moscow a few years earlier—an astounding and controversial feat for an American during the Cold War. Tickets to a Van Cliburn concert were hot items and probably expensive. Brian had no interest in classical music. He preferred cowboy songs: "Red River Valley," "Tumbling Tumbleweeds," "Back in the Saddle Again."

But he thought that as a budding pianist who had been taking piano lessons since age 7, *I* might be interested. He was right. Those Van Cliburn tickets taught me that the best gifts are chosen with the recipient firmly in mind. Buy what *they* like, not what you wish someone would give *you*.

Support and encourage young people

No one could make me feel as clever or as smart as Brian did. He gushed over the little curtains I sewed for his houseboat. He raved about the drum-shaped red, white, and blue cake I baked for a family 4th of July picnic. Knowing I didn't get an allowance and needed spending money in high school, he paid me to wash and iron his shirts, 50 cents each. Such an easy job. All his shirts were top-quality and almost wrinkle-free straight from the dryer.

Stick with a job

Brian was a meat cutter for a large grocery chain and personally selected every Thanksgiving turkey and Easter ham my mom baked, every steak my dad grilled. Standing on chilly, wet cement for long hours gave him cold feet for the rest of his life, but the work was steady, paid well, and offered benefits, so he stuck with it. Brian liked providing a service to shoppers feeding their families. He was good at it, and his stick-to-itiveness modeled a lesson for me: There's value in any job if you do your best.

Make people laugh

Brian cracked us up with his stories about difficult customers. Like the ones who rang the bell at the meat counter to ask for a special cut and, when he brought out their request, decided something already in the display case was what they wanted after all. That drove him crazy, though not quite as crazy as his stories would have you believe. He spun those tales to make us laugh.

Keep things neat

I shared a love of tidiness and minimalism with Brian. He was such a neatnik that family members joked if you slept in his guest room and got out of bed during the night to go to the bathroom, you'd come back to find he'd made your bed! For casual wear, he favored creased jeans, stored on hangers, and white tennis shoes. And I do mean white. Never a scuff mark. He purchased his favorite brand in bulk, stacking the boxes in his closet so he was always prepared to exchange soiled shoes for a pristine pair. He liked his teeth white, too, and bleached them to the point that one time, as he walked toward me from a distance, he looked like a beacon.

Brian enjoyed decorating, but he especially enjoyed *re*-decorating his suburban Detroit houses and condos. Out with the old and in with the new. Each home he owned was beautifully appointed in his thoughtful, spare style. He displayed only a few items: his pewter collection, a few wood carvings, some vases and bowls hand-blown by my brother. When my husband and I were poor graduate students, we were happy for the high-quality couches, tables, and chairs he passed on to us. Later, he thrilled my young daughter with a box of mini tart pans and pastry beans culled during one of his frequent kitchen cleanouts.

Stay fit

For his second-to-last home, Brian chose a split-level with lots of stairs. To keep his high blood pressure under control, he knew he needed to keep moving. To help resist late-night dessert, he brushed and flossed his teeth right after dinner. He and Russ loved to walk, several miles each day, on an ambitious circuit of errands—to the library, the bank, the produce market. They escaped Michigan winters by heading to Florida for vacations. And more walking. It's my favorite form of exercise, too.

***

After retiring, Brian continued to live his simple, quiet life with Russ. He read, took walks, watched television, spent time with family. I think he was happy. Or at least content.

When he started having trouble following conversations, a hearing aid seemed to help. Then one event changed everything: Russ collapsed on the bathroom floor. Brian covered him with a blanket and stayed alone inside the house without telling anyone what had happened. After the police carried Russ's body away, we found four days' worth of unopened Meals on Wheels boxes in the refrigerator.

With Russ's death came a revelation: he had been shielding the family from Brian's growing dementia, not wanting to "bother" us. Doctors diagnosed Alzheimer's disease.

Brian spent his last few years in a small memory care home, a place with worn, dated furnishings he definitely would not have approved of before dementia. But the home was clean, the care kind, the meals homemade. Brian won everyone over with his sweet disposition.

When I visited we drank Vernors, Brian's favorite soda, and popped sheets of bubble wrap to occupy his fidgety fingers. I tried to express how grateful I was to have him in my life. I thanked him for that Van Cliburn concert, for making me feel special, for taking my side during all those teenage arguments with my parents. In return, as always, he told stories that made me laugh.

I hated knowing that Brian was alone so much of the time. So, following his "Give good gifts" lesson, I bought him a robotic puppy we named Sandy. I showed him how to cup the dog's cheek to get it to nuzzle his hand, how to stroke the dog's back to activate a heartbeat sensation. Brian quickly warmed to Sandy. When he tugged on the puppy's bandana, it raised its eyebrows and wagged its tail. When he blew gently on Sandy's nose, the dog replied with a few soft barks. Best of all, Sandy didn't make a mess. A good gift for a neatnik.

About the Author: After a career as a librarian, Paulette Sharkey turned to writing. She is the author of dozens of articles for parents' and children's magazines, as well as a picture book, *A Doll for Grandma: A Story about Alzheimer's Disease*, illustrated by Samantha Woo (Beaming Books, 2020), inspired by her work as a volunteer pianist in memory care homes. All author proceeds from the sale of *A Doll for Grandma* support research to end Alzheimer's disease. Paulette lives with her husband in East Lansing, Michigan. You can follow Paulette on Twitter @pbsharkey or through her website http://paulettesharkey.com.

Cooking by Kindle Light
Sarah Veness

Sarah Veness was diagnosed with subcortical vascular dementia in 2011 but improved beyond her doctor's expectations. At 56-years-old she was rediagnosed with mild cognitive impairment following a head injury and a subsequent stroke. Sarah has remained stable and at 66, she is continuing to inspire and empower those she comes into contact with. She now lives in a supported living complex in the UK.

Mary Berry looked at me kindly with her steely blue eyes. "I have a foolproof way that will give you success every time and your problems will be over."

I wish! This was a reference to making meringues and not a cure for all of life's difficulties. I wanted to make a pavlova without the palaver.

My memory problems mean that cooking is quite a challenge as my executive functioning isn't all that it could be. I knew I was on dodgy ground when I looked in the fridge for a knife, even more so when I did it a second time in as many minutes.

Mary assured me that her tried and tested 'puds' stand the test of time. Painstakingly she breaks the eggs and I feel comforted as a piece of shell drops into the basin but they omit to show her scrabbling to get it out, which in my opinion would add a touch of realism to the proceedings. I like the fact that she is wearing a loom band bracelet probably made lovingly by a grandchild, it adds to the homey air of informality that she embodies.

To prove the consistency of the meringue she holds a spoonful above her head. I watch with bated breath wondering how many times they had to film the sequence and whether she ever got the thickness wrong. Heaven help us if I try and it cascades from the spoon, my hair becoming stiff and sticky as if it has been lacquered by an overzealous trainee hairdresser.

She shapes it into a perfect circle, makes a dip in the middle, and recreates the alps as she fluffs up small points around the edge and pops it in the oven for an hour.

I only put the cream in the top of my concoction and roughly chop up some strawberries and similar fruits and fling them on as the final touch. Mary mixes her berries with cassis liqueur and combines her fruits with a sugar syrup before she fills the cavity of her now cooled pavlova. Voila! Perfection!

Visiting my consultant he asked me how I was getting along with my cooking. I explained that it took me about three times as long as other people, involved quite a lot of charred dinners, and in the words of my mother "people just had to like it or lump it."

He said I'm not supposed to cook unsupervised but I do, but in our new kitchen, I feel more confident. I am sure he would be impressed with the professionals who I have chosen to accompany me on my gastronomic adventures. I am not alone in the kitchen anymore.

Next up is Nigella the culinary icon who said "it's probably quite relaxing for normal people to see a normal person like me cooking and making a mess and in a kitchen." That was reassuring, to say the least.

Her lemon pavlova with its billowy base, satiny peaks, and her reassuring honesty that patience isn't one of her outstanding qualities makes me drool as I watch her with her milk chocolate smooth voice and voluptuous presence.

It's never like that in my kitchen. My billows are more like tempestuous explosions of egg white than Nigella's, her meringue becomes glossier. She manages to finely grate the zest of a lemon without the added bit of fingernail in the mix or grazing her knuckles with the grater.

Smiling contentedly she uses the mixture on the whisk to make a glue in a moment of culinary creativity to stick the baking sheet to the cooking tray. Candles appear to flicker around her as she adores the snowy marshmallow spilling onto the sheet in all its alpine glory.

She may cook by candlelight but I cook by Kindle light. Her sensuous murmurings are replaced by my Essex girl vernacular as the egg white slops onto the tray. She flattens and smooths it into a circular shape which she finds rather restful whereas my flailing spatula struggles to make any recognisable form at all.

Thank goodness her pavlova cracks, which makes me feel marginally better. Having spread the top with lemon curd she then dollops on the cream and coaxes it to the edges with a long breathy emphasis on the word coaxes.

Wearing an elegant black dress with not a single grain of sugar on it and her hair bouncing and gleaming like a shampoo advert I look down and notice eggy finger marks on my jeans and my apron looks as if I've just returned from a war zone.

She goes on to explain slightly patronizingly how to toast your almonds "in a frying pan" as if I would attempt to brown mine in the toaster!

As she grates some more zest, her teeth sparkle between her lustrous lips and she can't wait to sink them into this lemony lusciousness. I can't wait to get my gnashers into mine either!

The final product looks marginally like hers, but only just. The proof of the pudding is in the eating!

The dodginess of my cooking continues as I try to put the olive oil into the Aga rather than into the cupboard.

Jamie Oliver is a whizz at Yorkshire puddings, needless to say, I am not. The cheeky boy with lots of chutzpah laughs as he invites us to make them perfectly. Hands cupped and eyes gleaming he throws a bowl into the air and catches it. With a wink and a whisk, he breaks the eggs single-handedly and beats the hell out of them. I need to break mine carefully into a cup first.

It's obviously all in the wrist action as he beats the batter and transfers it faultlessly into a jug ready for pouring. "Use a spoon as you put the mix into the tins so you don't splatter your batter," he says "as this will drag your

Yorkshires down, and we would never want that to happen."

He pops them into the oven with strict instructions not to open the oven door. Needless to say, I forget this tip, and having been rising like skyrockets they then sink to become Yorkshire pancakes. His crispy crunchy delights bear no similarity to my flat flabby failures.

Regarding the puddings at eye-level, words of delight spring from his lips and provoke me to feelings of envy and inferiority.

Next time I must keep replaying the video and not allow his cocky attitude to rub off, thinking I know what comes next because sadly I don't.

Yesterday I cooked spaghetti bolognese, I have no idea where the grape came from that appeared in the mix and even less of a clue as to how a rubber band materialised on one of the plates as I spooned the spaghetti out of the saucepan. It was the same colour and texture but fortunately was raw and I spotted it just before the pasta engulfed it.

It took my mind back to when I went to an aunt's house for tea and she gave me the skin off the custard. I knew this was Uncle Fred's favourite part of the pudding but she said, "What the eye doesn't see, the heart won't grieve over." It took years for me to understand what she meant.

My party piece is setting off the smoke and heat detectors which usually signifies dinner is ready! The noise makes your ears zing and you can feel the eardrums pulsating to an angry rhythm and of course, it mostly happens when people with extra sensitive hearing are in the house. I have never worked out why the heat detector remained silent when I set a frying pan of oil on fire.

I love being able to cook by Kindle light. There it rests on its little stand, propped up ready for me to spring into action, enhancing my skills and teaching me new ones. I never knew I had been cooking poached eggs wrongly for decades!

Backwards and forwards I go over the YouTube video clips, pausing, rewinding, replaying, refreshing my memory, creating old favourites, and attempting new challenges.

In the words of the fridge magnet, I need to "Keep calm and cook on" and I must take heart. After all many have eaten my cooking, and gone on to live healthy, productive lives!

About the Author: Sarah Veness is an award-winning author with mild cognitive impairment who is motivated by her own life events to encourage and inform people about dementia and memory issues. Written with compassion and humour, these stories appeal to those affected directly or indirectly by cognitive impairment, as well as those who enjoy a comforting read. She only discovered she enjoyed writing after her diagnosis.

Sarah's first book, *The Memory Box,* is available on Amazon in paperback, large print, and e-book. Bit.ly/sarahveness It includes her prize-winning story for the National Memory Day short story competition, run by the Alzheimer's Society.

Her second book *Phoebe's Feline Lowdown on Lockdown* is a humorous diary of lockdown told through the eyes of her cat Phoebe Furnackerpan. It is also available on Amazon as an e-book and paperback getbook.at/PFLL.

Inspired by the National Memory Day Creative Writing competition, Sarah is in the process of writing her third book, an anthology of short stories and poems based around the theme of memory. As someone who cares for a friend with early-onset Alzheimer's and also lives with memory loss herself, she hopes she can express the viewpoint of both caregivers and of those people who are in a position similar to her own.

Sarah has trained as a UK Dementia Champion and helps run a reminiscence group to affirm people's memories, called "I Remember It Well" and gives talks on how to make memory books and boxes. At 66 she is continuing to inspire people through her writing and as a motivational speaker and friend.

You can find Sarah here:
Twitter @creativesarahv
Facebook sarahveness.9
Email creativecardsbysarah@yahoo.co.uk
website (still in the making stage www.acatsatonic.co.uk)

Index of Authors

Alexander, Jan Morgan	89
Boreham, Elissa	103
	107
Bunt, Deb	61
Copeland-Parker, Tony	111
Corn, Donna	79
Doyle, Adam S	10
	149
Field, Steve	17
Fink, Jennifer	129
Galindo, Miriam	119
Green, Miriam	6
	8
Greenberg, Phyllis Joly	55
Harmon, MD, Renée Brown	82
Heins, Gincy	150
Hill, Grant	69
Klaeb, Melissa	92
Landeis, Susan	36
Lucas, Karla	79
Malena, Karen	96
McGuire, Teri Hayes	73

Miller, LeAnn Morgan	89
Nelson, Mary	77
Roberts, Patricia	28
Sciucco, Marianne	47
Sharkey, Paulette	134
Thelker, Christine	1
Veness, Sarah	140
White, Susanne	42
Wick, Annette Januzzi	20

About the Cover Art

Adam S Doyle's work is fueled by a love for the human mark. Since our ancestors smeared pigment on cave walls in the shape of wildlife millennia ago, humanity's legacy of asserting our existence is something built into being human. His work continues the tradition by keeping the stroke of paint visible.

Painting is also a transformation; the cave wall, the blank page, and the white canvas becomes a spacious place or a living, breathing being. He continues to be fascinated with this magical act. The unfinished quality to Doyle's work is about keeping this doorway between worlds partly open.

Nature and wildlife are primary subjects for both the connection he feels towards them and the diverse metaphorical language they afford in communicating ideas.

Doyle's father was an osteopathic physician who practiced Chinese medicine specializing in acupuncture for 50 years. Because of him the idea of energy flowing through our bodies has been in the artist's consciousness since childhood. Depicting energy is something he continues to explore in new directions, re-enchanting us with daily life.

The portrait of Dr. James Doyle was painted when Adam had the thought that his father might not be around forever. He had actually never painted his dad before. As it turned out, the expressive moment captured would reveal the truth of Adam's concern. Fortunately his father was around long enough to appreciate the gesture.

About Gincy Heins

Gincy Heins is the creator and editor of *Before the Diagnosis: Stories of Life and Love Before Dementia*, which contains 36 essays about individuals before their dementia diagnosis. She is also co-author of the *365 Caregiving Tips: Practical Tips from Everyday Caregivers* book series.

Gincy is the caregiver and advocate for her husband who was diagnosed with mild cognitive impairment when he was 55-years-old. She is also a mom, teacher, speaker, city commissioner, and volunteer with AlzAuthors and Alzheimer's Orange County. Gincy has been a speaker at several conferences including the Caregiver Smile Summit 3 and has been a guest on several podcasts. In Spring 2020, in order to help herself and others cope with the pandemic, Gincy posted daily videos on social media to spread a positive message each day.

You can connect with Gincy on Facebook (G-j Heins), Twitter (@GincyHeins) and Instagram (GincyHeins) and on her website, GincyHeins.com.

www.ingramcontent.com/pod-product-compliance
Lightning Source LLC
Chambersburg PA
CBHW071503220526
45472CB00003B/898